Otolar

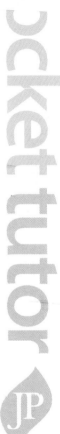

Otolaryngology

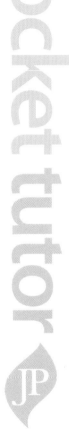

Abir Bhattacharyya MS FACS FRCS(Eng) FRCS(ORL)
Consultant ENT Surgeon and Royal College
Surgical Tutor
Associate Director of Medical Education (Surgery)
Whipps Cross University Hospital
London, UK

Nitesh Patel MBChB(Hons), FRCS(Eng), FRCS(ORL-HNS)
Consultant ENT Surgeon
Whipps Cross University Hospital
London, UK

medical
publishers

© 2012 JP Medical Ltd.

Published by JP Medical Ltd, 83 Victoria Street, London, SW1H 0HW, UK

Tel: +44 (0)20 3170 8910 Fax: +44 (0)20 3008 6180

Email: info@jpmedpub.com Web: www.jpmedpub.com

ISBN: 978-1-907816-11-6

British Library Cataloguing in Publication Data
A catalogue record for this book is available from the British Library

Library of Congress Cataloging in Publication Data
A catalog record for this book is available from the Library of Congress

JP Medical Ltd is a subsidiary of Jaypee Brothers Medical Publishers (P) Ltd, New Delhi, India

Publisher:	Richard Furn
Development Editor:	Paul Mayhew
Editorial Assistant:	Katrina Rimmer
Design:	Designers Collective Ltd
Index:	Liz Granger

Typeset, printed and bound in India.

Foreword

This pocket-sized book is the right size for the many doctors who encounter ENT disorders, whatever stage they have reached in their careers. Unfortunately exposure to ENT is now very variable and often sparse in undergraduate medical education in the UK, and yet the clinical relevance of ENT remains high for many doctors. Large numbers of patients present with ear nose or throat symptoms, particularly to GPs and paediatricians but also to many others. All doctors need to know something about the specialty because there are important life-threatening ENT conditions which can be missed or mismanaged with dire consequences – for instance, subdural empyema secondary to frontal sinusitis, meningitis secondary to acute otitis media and airway obstruction secondary to supraglottitis in adults.

This book is designed to be a comprehensive but portable resource that will prove a valuable aid to doctors of all grades. For those who work in ENT during their foundation years or as part of a rotation in basic training programmes it will prove particularly valuable. Clearly such readers should undergo an induction programme during their ENT exposure, but they will need access to more information when on call for ENT. With this book in their pocket or readily accessible in their departments, they will have rapid access to information and will be in a position to acquire valuable knowledge. The clinical scenarios should prove particularly useful in this setting.

Pocket Tutor Otolaryngology provides a lot of information in a useful accessible format. It will assist those who use it to make better decisions on patient management in real-life situations.

Alan Johnson
President
British Association of Otorhinolaryngologists,
Head and Neck Surgeons

Preface

When we were approached to write a pocket-size book on otolaryngology we were mindful of the challenges ahead. How to cover the breadth of a specialty that extends from 'dura to pleura'? How to incorporate the vast plethora of clinical information and ever-expanding knowledge that forms the basis of modern medical management? How to construct a concise yet trustworthy clinical tutor for your pocket?

In responding to this challenge we have tried to provide a conceptual framework for clinical thinking. The opening chapter, First Principles, explains the anatomical concepts and physiological principles that together form the building blocks for understanding normal and abnormal function. The second chapter, Clinical Essentials, summarises the examination techniques and investigative tools used to reach a diagnosis. The remaining chapters describe commonly seen clinical disorders. Since approximately one-third of patients seen in primary care have ENT-related pathology, we felt that brief clinical scenarios would be a simple and effective way of introducing a practical, evidence-based approach to the diagnosis and management of common presentations described in the clinical chapters. Another key feature is the 'clinical insight' and 'guiding principle' boxes interspersed within the text, which draw upon our personal experience.

Throughout the book, we have selected clinical topics which frequently present to the primary care practitioner, together with rare yet significant conditions which the medical student, trainee or junior doctor might encounter in the ward, outpatient clinic or emergency department of the hospital. Our selection is not exhaustive but we hope it is comprehensive for the intended audience.

We hope you will enjoy reading this book and that it will serve as a handy companion for quick reference thanks to its convenient pocket-size format. We shall be pleased to receive any comments, criticisms or suggestions at pockettutorotolaryngology@gmail.com.

Abir Bhattacharyya
Nitesh Patel
July 2011

Contents

Contributors

We offer our sincere gratitude to the following people who have made a significant contribution to this book.

ENT Consultants
Mr Furrat Amen, Mr Mriganka De

ENT Specialist Registrars

Jay Ahmed

Zaid Awad

Raghav Dwivedi

Behrad Elmiyah

Nancy Grover

Sanjeev Gupta

Rebecca Heywood

Elina Kiverniti

Elias Koury

Jai Manickavasaram

Serge Pal

Vyas Prasad

Baskaran Ranganathan

Anita Sonsale

Sarju Varsani

Vik Veer

Acknowledgements

Thanks to Julian East, Medical Photography Unit of Whipps Cross University Hospital, and Dr Cheng for helping with clinical photographs, often at very short notice. Thanks to the many GPs who have given written and verbal feedback to improve the manuscript. The list is long and we apologise for not being able to individually acknowledge all our primary care colleagues but we need to mention Dr A Dhanji, Dr S Dadabhoy and Dr I Bhatnagar for their suggestions.

Thanks also to JP Medical Publishers Ltd for their help and support. In particular we thank Paul Mayhew and Richard Furn for their constant encouragement.

Last but not least we acknowledge our families' sacrifice in letting us burn the midnight oil and work at weekends when deadlines were near. Abir would like to thank his wife (Rinku) and his children (Anudeep and Amrita) for letting him complete his academic work unhindered. Nitesh would like to thank Krishna, his mother, his wife (Hema) and his children (Seeta and Sai).

Abir Bhattacharyya
Nitesh Patel

First principles

1.1 Anatomy

Anatomy of the ear

The basic anatomy of the ear is shown in **Figure 1.1**. The ear is divided anatomically into **outer**, **middle** and **inner** sections, with the latter two embedded in the **temporal bone**. The sections contain the following structures:

- Outer ear: pinna, concha, and external auditory canal (EAC) or meatus
- Middle ear: tympanic membrane, tympanic cavity (or middle ear space), the three ossicles (malleus, incus and stapes), two muscles (stapedius and tensor tympani), a section of the chorda tympani nerve (a branch of the facial nerve) that passes through and the superior opening of the Eustachian tube
- Inner ear: the cochlea, vestibule and three semicircular canals.

Embryology

The external ear develops from six tubercles of the first branchial arch, as do the malleus, incus and tensor tympani. The stapes

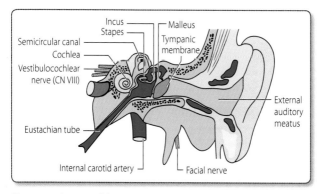

Figure 1.1 Anatomy of the ear.

Clinical insight

Failure of fusion of the six tubercles during embryological development can result in preauricular abnormalities (usually a sinus) or accessory auricles.

Clinical insight

- The cartilage of the pinna is entirely dependent on the closely adherent perichondrium for its blood supply. Any disruption between these layers, as with accumulations of blood or pus (haematoma or abscess), can result in avascular necrosis of the cartilage with cauliflower ear deformity
- The skin of the medial aspect of the EAC is thin, adherent and sensitive, so acute infection usually gives rise to excruciating pain.

and stapedius are derived from the second arch (**Figure 1.2**). The distal portion of the first pharyngeal pouch comes into contact with the epithelial lining of the first pharyngeal cleft, forming the **EAC**; the proximal portion of the first pharyngeal pouch forms the middle ear and the Eustachian (or pharyngotympanic) tube.

The tympanic membrane is formed from an ectodermal epithelial lining, an intermediate layer of mesenchyme and an endodermal lining from the first pharyngeal pouch.

The inner ear develops from the **otic vesicle**, an epithelial sac derived from the surface ectoderm of the neural tube.

The external ear and acoustic meatus

The external ear or **pinna** is cartilaginous with closely adherent perichondrium. The blood supply of the cartilage of the pinna is entirely dependent on the perichondrium. The EAC (**Figure 1.3**) is about 25 mm in length, cartilaginous in the outer one third and bony in the inner two thirds.

Wax is made up of secretions produced from specialised sweat glands in the EAC called **ceruminous glands**, and skin cells. Skin and wax usually migrate radially outward from the tympanic membrane and then laterally along the EAC.

The tympanic membrane

The **tympanic membrane** (eardrum) is composed of three layers (skin, fibrous tissue and mucosa), in keeping with its

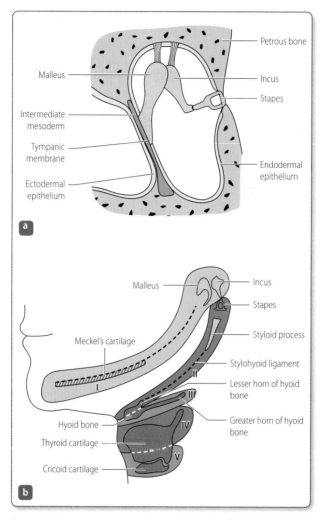

Figure 1.2 Derivation of the tympanic membrane (a) and structures derived from the pharyngeal arches (b).

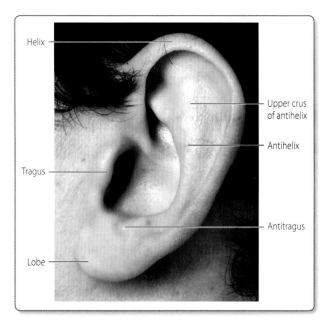

Helix

Upper crus
of antihelix

Antihelix

Tragus

Antitragus

Lobe

Figure 1.3 The pinna.

embryological origin. The normal appearance is pearly and opaque and its slight concavity results in the '**light reflex**' (**Figure 1.4**), a characteristic triangular cone of light seen when light is reflected from its surface.

The **pars tensa** is the larger inferior section of the membrane and has a well-organised fibrous (middle) layer and an annulus or thickened ring at the periphery. In the smaller superior portion, the **pars flaccida**, the fibrous middle layer is poorly organised and the annulus is incomplete superiorly.

The middle ear

The **middle ear** (**Figure 1.5**) is an air-containing space, and developmentally a continuation of the Eustachian tube. It contains three small middle ear bones called **ossicles** – the **malleus**, **incus** and **stapes**. The **tensor tympani** attaches the

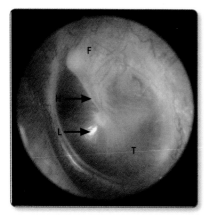

Figure 1.4 Left tympanic membrane. F, pars flaccida; H, handle of malleus; L, light reflex; T, pars tensa.

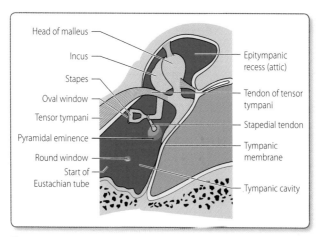

Figure 1.5 Middle ear anatomy

malleus to cartilage of the Eustachian tube and dampens background sounds such as chewing. The 1 mm long **stapedius** muscle attaches the neck of the stapes to the pyramidal eminence of the posterior middle ear wall and prevents loud sounds causing acoustic trauma. It also functions reflexively to dampen background low frequency sound such as the sound of one's own voice. The round and oval windows, lateral semicircular canal, basal turn of the cochlea and tympanic plexus of nerves are closely related to the medial aspect of the middle ear.

Temporal bone The pneumatised (air-filled) mastoid cells in the temporal bone are connected to the middle ear through the aditus. This reservoir of air helps prevent wide fluctuations of middle ear pressure. Chronic middle ear disease reduces the pneumatisation, causing a sclerotic (dense) mastoid.

The facial nerve The facial nerve has a long and tortuous course through the temporal bone, exiting through the stylo-mastoid foramen in front of the mastoid process (see p. 88 for more anatomy of the facial nerve).

The facial nerve controls the motor activity of most facial muscles, and it has intimate association with the middle and inner ear after it courses through the internal auditory canal in the petrous part of the temporal bone. It also contains sensory afferents, including the **chorda tympani**, which carries taste fibres from the anterior two thirds of the tongue. The facial nerve is posterosuperior to the medial wall of the middle ear.

Clinical insight

The chorda tympani is susceptible to damage in chronic middle ear conditions and surgeries. In taste it appears to inhibit other sensory signals (e.g. from the glossopharyngeal nerve), therefore damage causes erratic changes in taste rather than a loss of sensation.

The Eustachian tube The Eustachian tube extends from the anterior wall of the middle ear to the lateral wall of the nasopharynx. About one third of the tube proximal to the middle ear is bony; the rest is composed of cartilage and the base raises a tubal eleva-tion, the torus tubarius, which opens into the nasopharynx. The tube is shorter, wider and more horizontal in children, making them more prone to middle ear infections than adults. The opening of the tube during swallowing, with the action of the muscles of the palate, allows aeration of the middle ear and the equalising of pressures either side of the tympanic membrane.

The inner ear

The inner ear consists of:

- the vestibule and semicircular canals, responsible
  for balance
- the cochlea, responsible
  for hearing.

Clinical insight

Eustachian tube blockage due to adenoidal hypertrophy or neoplasm prevents adequate middle ear aeration, and fluid may accumulate in the middle ear causing deafness.

They lie within a bony labyrinth (network of canals), which is one of the densest bones in the body and protects the closely adjacent membranous labyrinth and its sensitive neuroepithelium. The membranous labyrinth is hollow and filled with **endolymph**, a fluid with similar ionic concentrations to intracellular fluid. **Perilymph,** surrounding the membranous labyrinth, is a filtrate of blood and cerebrospinal fluid (CSF) and is similar to extracellular fluid. The endolymph transmits vibrations to the membranes via electromechanically sensitive cells called **hair cells** which generate action potentials subsequently transmitted to the vestibulocochlear nerve (cranial nerve VIII).

The vestibule The vestibule is the 'entrance' to the inner ear, via its oval window on the lateral (tympanic) wall, and measures 5 x 5 x 3 mm. It sits behind the cochlea and in front of the semicircular canals and consists of two membranous sacs: the saccule and the utricle. It contains receptors that sense gravity and acceleration.

The cochlea The snail-shaped cochlea is a system of 3 tubes coiled 2.5 turns and a bony core called the **modiolus**. It contains the cochlear duct of the membranous labyrinth, which has a pair of perilymph filled chambers, the scala vestibuli and the scala tympani either side (**Figure 1.6**). Inside the cochlear duct, in a structure known as the organ of Corti, there are nearly 20 000 hair cells, each connecting to its own nerve receptor. These are stimulated by endolymph movement generated by the footplate of the stapes at the oval window. The movement of endolymph is sensed by the stereocilia of the inner and outer hair cells.

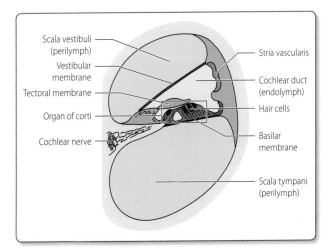

Figure 1.6 Cross section of the cochlea

The semicircular canals The three semicircular canals (superior, posterior and lateral) are at right angles to each other. Each canal has a widening called the ampulla which contains the embedded neuroepithelial hair cells. Rotatory motion, linear acceleration and deceleration result in movement of the surrounding endolymph and corresponding movement of the hair cells – the vestibular inputs are integrated with proprioceptive and visual inputs in the brainstem to maintain balance.

The auditory pathway The auditory pathway from the cochlea to the cortex, with processing occurring at each stage, can be summarised as:
- Cochlear (or auditory) nerve
- Cochlear nuclei of the pons and medulla oblongata
- Superior olivary nucleus of the brainstem (mostly pontine)
- Inferior colliculus of the midbrain
- Medial geniculate nucleus of the thalamus
- Auditory cortex of the temporal lobe.

The vestibular pathway The vestibular pathway is responsible for balance and co-ordinates movement perception with postural muscle tone (see 'Physiology of balance', p. 27):
- Vestibular nerve
- Four vestibular nuclei of medulla (and pons)
- Branches to eye muscle nuclei:
  - CN III (oculomotor nerve innervating medial rectus)
  - CN VI (abducens nerve innervating lateral rectus)
- Branches to vestibulospinal tract (head and trunk movement co-ordination)
- Branches to cerebellum.

Anatomy of the nose

The external nose consists of a bony and mainly cartilaginous skeleton (**Figure 1.7**). The two nasal cavities are separated by a bony and cartilaginous septum and terminate at the posterior **choanae** (from the Greek word for funnel), which lead to the nasopharynx.

The nasal vestibule is the most anterior part of the nose. Each is formed by nasal cartilages, connective tissue and hair-bearing skin. The main cartilages are the bilateral greater alar cartilages (lower lateral cartilages) and the cartilaginous nasal septum.

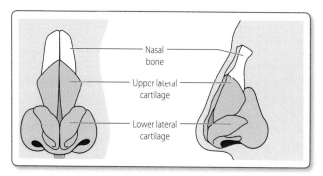

Nasal bone

Upper lateral cartilage

Lower lateral cartilage

Figure 1.7 Cartilaginous skeleton of the nose.

The junction between the nasal vestibule and the nasal cavity is the narrowest part of the nasal airway, known as the internal nasal valve.

Lateral nasal wall On the lateral wall of the nose are three turbinates (inferior, middle and superior) or bony ridges which increase the surface area of the nasal mucosa; they have a rich nerve and blood supply, and are therefore sensate. The ostia (openings) of the sinuses, apart from the sphenoid sinus and the opening of the nasolacrimal duct, are located on the lateral wall of the nose in the meatus that lie inferior to the turbinates (**Table 1.1**).

Blood supply of the medial nasal wall Little's area is an anterioinferior part of the nasal septum where four arteries meet to form Kiesselbach's plexus. This is a rich vascular anastomosis between the internal and external carotid artery systems (**Figure 1.8**).

Paranasal sinuses

The paranasal sinuses (**Figure 1.9**) are divided into groups named according to the bones in which they lie:

Meatus	Sinus ostia
Superior	Opening of the posterior ethmoidal sinus
Middle	• All open into the hiatus semilunaris: • Anterior ethmoidal sinuses • Frontal sinus through the frontonasal recess • Maxillary sinus
Inferior	Opening of the nasolacrimal duct

Table 1.1 Lateral nasal wall – meatus and sinus ostia (openings)

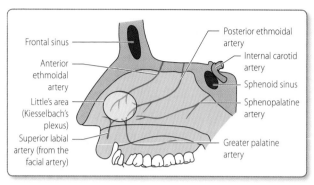

Figure 1.8 Blood supply of the medial wall of the nose.

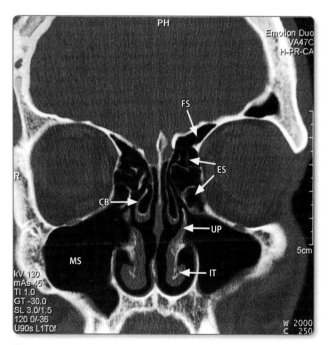

Figure 1.9 Paranasal sinuses. Frontal sinus (FS); ethmoid sinuses (ES); uncinate process (UP); inferior turbinate (IT); concha bullosa (CB); maxillary sinus (MS).

- The **maxillary sinuses** (or antra) are the largest of the paranasal sinuses and are located in the maxillary bones. The superior wall is the floor of the orbit, the sinus floor is formed by the alveolar process of the maxilla and can sometimes be perforated by the apices of the molar teeth. This sinus can be involved in orbital blowout fracture and root canal and dental infections
- The **frontal sinus** in the frontal bone, superior to the eyes, forms the roof of the orbit; its posterior wall is the bony anterior cranial fossa
- The **ethmoid sinuses** are formed from several discrete air cells within the ethmoid bone between the nose and the eyes. They are further divided according to their drainage into anterior and posterior groups (**Table 1.1**). The lateral wall forms the (paper-thin) **lamina papyracea**, which separates the sinus from the orbital cavity. Ethmoidal infection, especially in children but also in adults, can breach the lamina and involve the orbit, with the potential to affect vision by compressing the orbital contents
- The **sphenoid sinuses** are in the sphenoid bone at the centre of the skull base under the pituitary gland. The lateral walls are related to vital structures, including the internal carotid artery, cavernous sinus and cranial nerves II–IV. The transnasal approach to the pituitary gland is through the sphenoid sinuses.

Anatomy of the head and neck
The neck
The neck contains various layers of fascia that divide it into different compartments:
- **investing fascia** is the outermost layer just deep to the platysma
- **prevertebral fascia** is in front of the prevertebral muscles
- **pretracheal fascia** encloses the thyroid gland and allows gliding movement during swallowing

- the **carotid sheath** envelopes the common carotid artery, internal jugular vein and vagus nerve.

The neck is anatomically divided into anterior and posterior triangles and extends from the skull base above to the upper border of the sternum below.

Anterior triangle of the neck   The boundaries of the anterior triangle (**Figure 1.10**) are:

- Medial: midline of the neck from the chin to the manubrium sterni
- Lateral: anterior border of the sternocleidomastoid (as described by anatomists although surgeons clinically use the posterior border of sternocleidomastoid muscle)
- Superior: the lower border of the body of the mandible

The anterior neck is subdivided into four smaller triangles by the digastric muscle above and the superior belly of the omohyoid below. These four smaller triangles contain the following structures:

- The **muscular triangle**: the anterior neck muscles, larynx, thyroid, trachea and oesophagus

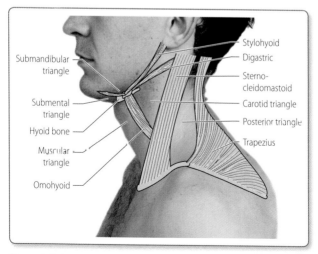

Figure 1.10 Triangles of the neck.

- The **carotid triangle:** the carotid sheath
- The **submandibular triangle** or **digastric triangle:** the submandibular gland, facial artery and vein, hypoglossal nerve, hypoglossus, mylohyoid muscle and nerve and glossopharyngeal nerve
- The **submental triangle:** the submental lymph nodes and anterior jugular vein.

Posterior triangle of the neck The posterior triangle contains the accessory nerve, the inferior belly of the omohyoid, the occipital artery, the external jugular vein, the lymph nodes and the cutaneous branch of the cervical plexus.

The floor is formed by the prevertebral fascia overlying the prevertebral muscles. Its boundaries are:
- Anterior: posterior border of the sternocleidomastoid muscle
- Posterior: anterior edge of the trapezius muscle
- Inferior: the middle third of the clavicle

Anatomical levels of the neck The anatomical landmarks of the triangles are subdivided into levels I–VI for oncological purposes (known as the Memorial Sloan–Kettering group). These are listed in **Table 1.2** and shown in **Figure 1.11**.

Level	Description
Ia	Submental (between anterior belly of digastric and neck midline)
Ib	Submandibular (bounded by anterior and posterior belly of digastric)
II	Between skull base and hyoid: below posterior belly of digastric (IIa); posterior to spinal accessory nerve (IIb)
III	Level of carotid bifurcation and omohyoid
IV	Between omohyoid and clavicle
V	Posterior triangle – between posterior border of sternocleidomastoid and anterior boundary of trapezius
VI	Anterior central compartment

Table 1.2 Anatomical levels of the neck

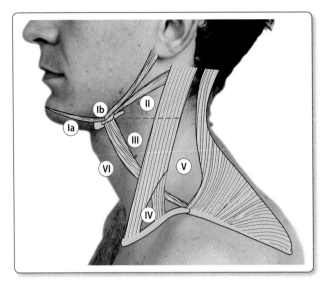

Figure 1.11 Anatomical levels of the neck.

Neck spaces and applied anatomy There are five neck spaces, as described below.

Parapharyngeal space This is an inverted pyramidal space formed above by the base of the skull and the petrous temporal bone, with its apex below at the hyoid bone. Infection can spread from the tonsils (quinsy), pharynx, teeth or salivary glands into this space and present with:

- Medial displacement of the lateral pharyngeal wall
- Potential airway obstruction
- Trismus, the inability to open the mouth
- Dysphagia, a difficulty swallowing
- Retromandibular fullness.

Potential complications include septic thrombosis of the internal jugular vein and airway obstruction.

Submandibular space This is a space in continuity with the floor of the mouth along the posterior edge of the mylohyoid.

The source of infection affecting this space is usually dental. The presenting features of infection or cellulitis (Ludwig's angina) are:

- Odynophagia, painful swallowing
- The feeling of being strangled
- Stridor and dyspnoea in severe cases.

Complications of Ludwig's angina involve the spread of infection via fascial planes, which leads to swelling and displacement of the tongue posteriorly and superiorly, causing airway compromise. It is a surgical emergency to drain the abscess and secure the airway.

Carotid sheath space   This is an area between the layers of fascia surrounding the neurovascular bundle – the carotid artery, internal jugular vein, vagus nerve and ansa cervicalis (a nerve loop that supplies the infrahyoid muscles). Infection is usually from the parapharyngeal or submandibular space, and the presenting feature is painful torticollis (a stiff, usually laterally flexed neck). Life-threatening complications such as septic shock, endocarditis and cavernous sinus thrombosis can result.

Pretracheal space   This is the space around the trachea, containing the pharynx, trachea, thyroid gland and oesophagus. Infection from the tonsils, trachea, oesophagus, or thyroid, or blunt laryngeal trauma, can present with:

- Odynophagia
- Hoarseness
- Emphysema (in some patients).

Complications include potential spread of infection to the mediastinum, mediastinal emphysema, and laryngeal oedema.

Retropharyngeal space   This space behind the pharynx and oesophagus contains lymph nodes, the greatest numbers of which are found in children under the age of 4. Infection from acute respiratory infections present with:

- Odynophagia
- Drooling
- Cervical rigidity
- *'Hot potato' voice*, where the patient speaks as if they have a mouthful of hot food.

Complications include pharyngeal swelling and abscess, with potential spread to the mediastinum, airway obstruction and rupture of abscess causing aspiration pneumonia.

Pharynx and oral cavity

The boundaries and relationships of the pharynx and oral cavity are shown in **Figure 1.12**.

Nasopharynx This is bound superiorly by the skull base and inferiorly by an imaginary line level with the soft palate. Anteriorly are the posterior choanae and laterally the Eustachian tube openings. The posterior nasopharynx contains pharyngeal mucosa and, in children, adenoid tissue.

Oropharynx This extends from the level of the soft palate to the base of the valeculla, i.e. the level of the hyoid bone. It contains the palatine tonsils bilaterally.

Hypopharynx (laryngopharynx) This extends from the base of the valeculla to the inferior edge of the cricoid cartilage. It has subdivisions of the posterior pharyngeal wall, post-cricoid region and pyriform fossae.

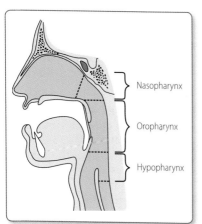

Figure 1.12 Boundaries: nasopharynx, oropharynx and hypopharynx.

Clinical insight

Killian's dehiscence is a potential weakness between the two divisions of the inferior constrictor muscle: the thyropharyngeus above and the cricopharyngeus below. A pharyngeal pouch (see p. 183) is a herniation of the posterior pharyngeal mucosa through the dehiscence.

Larynx and trachea

The larynx or 'voice box' has a cartilaginous skeleton consisting of three single (thyroid, cricoid and epiglottic) and three paired (arytenoid, corniculate and cuneiform) cartilages (**Figure 1.13**). The larynx extends vertically from the tip of the epiglottis to the inferior border of the cricoid cartilage – the only complete cartilaginous ring above the trachea. Its interior can be divided into the:

- **Supraglottis**: consisting of the whole epiglottis, aryepiglottic folds, vestibular folds, ventricles and arytenoids
- **Glottis**: the vocal folds and the area 1 cm inferior to them
- **Subglottis**: below the glottis to the lower border of the cricoid cartilage.

Functionally, the larynx is essential in breathing, phonation and protecting the airways against aspiration.

Vocal folds The vocal folds (or cords) (**Figure 1.13**) are the only part of the larynx lined (superiorly) by stratified squamous epithelium; the rest of the respiratory tract is lined by pseudostratified ciliated columnar epithelium. The layered anatomy of the vocal folds is crucial to the physiology of phonation. The epithelial layer vibrates or glides over a loose layer of superficial lamina propria (Reinke's space) supported by a firm body (vocalis/thyroarytenoid muscle).

Nerve supply The internal branch of the superior laryngeal nerve supplies sensory innervation to the glottis and larynx above this level. The external branch of the superior laryngeal nerve is motor and supplies the cricothyroid muscle. The bilateral recurrent laryngeal nerves supply sensory innervation to the

Clinical insight

The lymphatic drainage of the glottis is poor compared to that of the supraglottis and pharynx, hence glottal tumours spread late and present early, with hoarse voice as an early symptom.

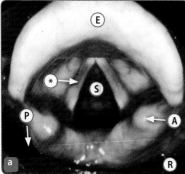

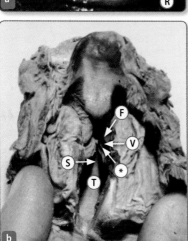

Figure 1.13 Vocal fold and laryngeal anatomy. (a) Endoscopic view of the larynx from above with the vocal folds in abduction (opened position). The trachea and subglottis are visualised through the rima glottidis. (b) Vertical cross-section through the larynx showing the false vocal folds, true vocal folds and the ventricles. A, arytenoid cartilage; E, epiglottis; F, false vocal fold; P, pyriform fossa; *, true vocal fold; R, right side; S, subglottis; T, trachea; V, ventricle.

subglottis and motor innervation to the rest of the pairs of intrinsic muscles of the larynx:

- Posterior cricoarytenoids (the only abductors)
- Lateral cricoarytenoids
- Transverse arytenoids
- Thyroarytenoids.

The course of each recurrent laryngeal nerve is long: the left recurrent laryngeal nerve loops around the aortic arch and travels in the tracheo-oesophageal groove; the right recurrent laryngeal nerve passes under the right subclavian artery and then upwards into the tracheo-oesophageal groove. Both enter the larynx at the **inferior cornu** of the thyroid cartilage.

Thyroid and parathyroid glands

Embryology The thyroid gland descends from the foramen caecum in the tongue base to its final position in front of the trachea. The thyroglossal duct normally involutes completely, however a thyroglossal cyst (see section 6.4) can develop anywhere along the duct, most commonly below the hyoid bone in the midline.

Anatomy The thyroid gland is a butterfly-shaped bilobed gland with a strand of thyroid tissue connecting the lobes called the isthmus. The gland is surrounded by its own capsule and pretracheal fascia. Between the two layers of the capsule or just outside the posterior side of the lobes are the superior (arising from the fourth pharyngeal pouch) and inferior (arising from the third pharyngeal pouch) parathyroid glands. The firm attachment of the thyroid gland to the underlying pretracheal fascia means that it moves during swallowing.

Neurovascular supply and lymphatic drainage The thyroid is supplied by the superior thyroid artery, a branch of the external carotid artery; the inferior thyroid artery, a branch of the thyrocervical trunk and in less than 10% of the population the thyroid ima artery, a branching directly from the brachiocephalic trunk. The recurrent laryngeal nerve and the inferior thyroid artery are closely related to the inferior pole of the gland and meticulous and careful dissection is required to avoid injury to the nerve during thyroid surgery. Lymphatic drainage frequently passes to the lateral deep cervical lymph nodes and the pre- and paratracheal lymph nodes.

Cranial nerves

The sensory and motor nerve supply to the ear, nose and throat is from the cranial nerves, which are summarised in **Table 1.3**. Testing of cranial nerve function is described in Chapter 2.

1.2 Physiology

Physiology of hearing

Sound is a mechanical vibration which sets up oscillations of air molecules. The ear is structured to collect, amplify and transduce this mechanical energy into action potentials. Signals generated in the cochlea travel to the cochlear nuclei of the brainstem via the auditory nerve; from the nuclei they branch to the thalamus and then on to the auditory cortex of the temporal lobes.

Outer ear

The external ear acts as a 'collecting device' for these vibrations and propagates the sound towards the tympanic membrane. The conchae and the EAC act as acoustic resonators, affecting the sound pressure at the tympanic membrane. The EAC contributes substantially to an increase in sound pressure level at the tympanic membrane. Pressure changes in the EAC vibrate the tympanic membrane, which in turn causes movement of the ossicular chain in the middle ear.

Nerve	Name	Sensory, motor or both	Origin	Nuclei	Foramina	Function
I	Olfactory	Purely sensory	Telencephalon	Anterior olfactory nucleus	Cribriform plate	**Sensory:** smell
II	Optic	Purely sensory	Diencephalon	Ganglion cells of retina	Optic canal	**Sensory:** sight
III	Oculomotor	Mainly motor	Anterior aspect of midbrain	Oculomotor nucleus, Edinger–Westphal nucleus	Superior orbital fissure	**Motor:** levator palpebrae superioris, all extraocular muscles (except superior oblique and lateral rectus), ciliary body and sphincter papillae
IV	Trochlear	Mainly motor	Dorsal aspect of midbrain	Trochlear nucleus	Superior orbital fissure	**Motor:** superior oblique muscle
V	Trigeminal: Ophthalmic – V_1 Maxillary – V_2 Mandibular – V_3	Both sensory and motor	Pons	Trigeminal nuclei: principal sensory, spinal, mesencephalic and motor	Superior orbital fissure – V_1 Foramen rotundum – V_2 Foramen ovale – V_3	**Motor:** muscles of mastication **Sensory:** face (largest cranial nerve)
VI	Abducens	Mainly motor	Posterior margin of pons	Abducens nucleus	Superior orbital fissure	**Motor:** lateral rectus (longest intracranial course)
VII	Facial	Both sensory and motor	Pons (cerebellopontine angle) above olive	Facial nucleus, solitary nucleus, superior salivary nucleus	Enters the internal acoustic canal and exits through stylomastoid foramen	**Motor:** muscles of facial expression, posterior belly of digastricus muscle, stapedius **Secretomotor:** salivary glands (except parotid) and lacrimal glands

Contd...

			Origin	Nuclei	Foramen	Function
						Sensory: taste from the anterior two thirds of tongue
VIII	Vestibulocochlear	Mostly sensory	Lateral to CN VII (cerebellopontine angle)	Vestibular nuclei, cochlear nuclei	Internal acoustic canal	**Sensory**: sound (cochlear), rotation and gravity (vestibular)
IX	Glossopharyngeal	Both sensory and motor	Medulla	Nucleus ambiguus, inferior salivary nucleus, solitary nucleus	Jugular foramen	**Motor**: stylopharyngeus **Secretomotor**: parotid gland **Sensory**: taste from the posterior third of the tongue
X	Vagus	Both sensory and motor	Posterolateral sulcus of medulla	Nucleus ambiguus, dorsal motor vagal nucleus, solitary nucleus	Jugular foramen	**Sensory**: EAC and posterior auricle; taste from epiglottis **Motor**: most laryngeal and all pharyngeal muscles (except stylopharyngeus) **Parasympathetic**: to nearly all thoracic and abdominal viscera
XI	Accessory nerve	Mainly motor	Cranial and spinal roots	Nucleus ambiguus, spinal accessory nucleus	Jugular foramen	**Motor**: sternocleidomastoid and trapezius muscles
XII	Hypoglossal nerve	Mainly motor	Medulla	Hypoglossal nucleus	Hypoglossal canal	**Motor:** tongue (except for the palatoglossus [XI])

CN, cranial nerve; EAC, external auditory canal.

Table 1.3 Cranial nerves: origin nuclei, foramina and function

Clinical insight

Middle ear conditions such as effusion, pressure changes and ossicular fixation increase its impedance, i.e. the opposition of motion subjected to force; this interferes with the transfer of sound energy. A useful measure of middle ear integrity can be provided by tympanometry, an objective measure of middle ear function (see section 2.4).

Middle ear

The middle ear is both a *coupler* (transferring sound from air to fluid media) and a *transformer* (the three ossicles increase the sound energy transmitted to the cochlea to a greater extent than would occur from a direct coupling). The movement of the tympanic membrane results in a focused application of force by the ossicular chain at the oval window. The piston-like vibration of the stapes in the oval window leads to a pressure differential between the scala vestibuli and the scala tympani, which is essential to the mechanical excitation of the cochlear hair cells. The transformer effect of the middle ear is primarily due to:

- The area of the tympanic membrane being greater than the area of the stapes footplate (**Figure 1.14**), which effectively allows 14 times the pressure at the footplate
- A lever system (**Figure 1.15**), whereby the displacement of the incus is less than that of the malleus, resulting in a greater application of force by ratio of 1.3:1.0.

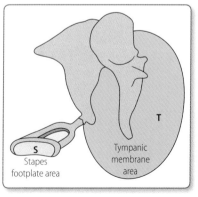

Figure 1.14 The ratio of the area of the tympanic membrane and stapes footplate (T/S) results in pressure increase at oval window.

T

S
Stapes footplate area

Tympanic membrane area

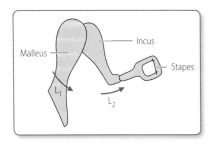

Figure 1.15 Unequal displacements of malleus (L_1) and incus (L_2) result in a pressure increase.

The acoustic reflex Stapedius has a protective role by reducing the intensity of sound signals reaching the inner ear, called the *acoustic* (or *attenuation*) *reflex*. When high intensity sound is transmitted to the cochlear nuclei of the brainstem, interneurons to the pontine motor nuclei of the facial nerve initiate a reflex after just 40–80 ms:

- Stapedius (innervated by the facial nerve) contracts to pull the stapes away from the oval window of the cochlea
- The physiology of the human tensor tympani remains obscure. In contrast to findings in most animals, it does not respond to sound unless the sound is strong, sudden and causes a 'startle' response.

The sum effect is to make the ossicular chain rigid, thereby attenuating transmission of lower frequency sound by up to 40 dB. Sounds of long duration are suppressed at high levels, whereas short-duration bursts of sound energy are transmitted relatively unimpeded by middle ear muscle activity. This attenuation is also initiated pre-emptively, such as just before speaking.

Inner ear

Displacement of perilymph within the scala vestibuli by the motion of the stapes imparts a travelling wave of vibration to the **basilar membrane** (**Figure 1.6**) of the cochlear duct. The travelling wave builds up to a maximum depending on the pitch, and then falls to nothing. The wave peaks near the base of the cochlea for high-pitched sounds (where it is stiffer), and near the apex for low-pitched sounds. The fluid wave causes a shearing force on the **stereocilia** of the hair cells that bends them and induces a receptor potential (**Figure 1.16**). This causes the release of neurotransmitters. There are two types of hair cell:

- **inner hair cells** are responsible for the majority of the acoustic nerve signal
- **outer hair cells** *amplify* sound-induced vibrations by vibrating at the frequency of the acoustic signal (known as *mechanical feedback amplification*).

Neurotransmitters released at the base of the hair cell generate excitatory post-synaptic potentials (EPSPs) in primary afferent nerve fibres of the auditory nerve. All-or-nothing responses propagate through these axons to second-order fibres in the brainstem. About one fifth of a second after detection,

> ## Clinical insight
>
> In the healthy cochlea vibration of the outer hair cells in response to noise generates acoustic energy, known as *otoacoustic emissions* (OAEs). This principle is utilised in screening the hearing of newborn babies. A probe is placed in the EAC and generates wideband clicks. Acoustic energy produced in response to the clicks is detected by a microphone within the probe. Automated OAE screeners display the results of the test as either *pass* or *refer*.

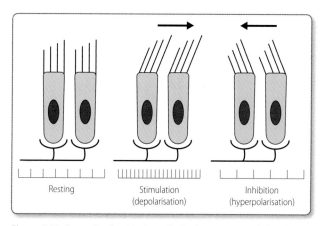

Figure 1.16 Stereocilia of cochlea hair cells. Displacement towards the tallest row of stereocilia is depolarising.

electrical signals reach the auditory cortex of the temporal lobes and sounds are perceived.

Cells in the central auditory system are exquisitely sensitive to small differences in intensity and time differences of the sound arriving at both ears, giving rise to the ability to localise sound.

Physiology of balance

Balance is maintained by co-ordination of information from three main sensory systems (**Figure 1.17**):

- The vestibular system
- The eyes
- Proprioception, i.e. sensory information from muscles, joints, tendons and ligaments.

The signals from these systems are integrated in the brainstem, cerebellum and cortex. Disorders affecting any of these structures or their physiology (e.g. cardiac, respiratory, metabolic diseases) can affect balance.

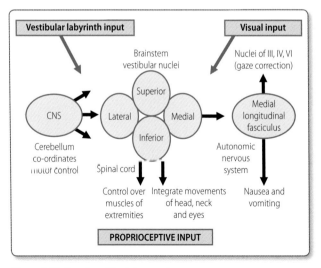

Figure 1.17 Overview of the balance system.

Vestibular system

Vestibular labyrinth In the inner ear the vestibular labyrinth detects acceleration of the head in any direction, whether in a straight line (linear) or turning (angular). Similar to the cochlear system of sensing hearing, the mechanical stimuli are transduced into electrical impulses which travel along the vestibular nerve to the brainstem.

Utricle and saccule The utricle and saccule of the vestibule are called the **otolithic** organs: they contain crystals surrounded by less dense endolymph. The difference in flow response of the crystals and endolymph is sensed by hair cells during linear acceleration (**Figure 1.18**), such as side-to-side or up-and-down movement. When the head is tilted from side to side, gravity will cause a shearing force between the otolithic membrane and the surface of the maculae, resulting in a bending of the stereocilia. The deflection of the stereocilia in the direction of the longer stereocilia causes the transduction channels to open, allowing hair cell depolarisation. Conversely, movement of the stereocilia in the opposite direction causes hyperpolarisation. The hair cells then generate vestibular nerve action potentials, which sends information about head position to the brainstem and spinal cord. This is relayed to eye muscles (utricle) and posture muscles (saccule).

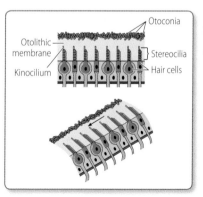

Figure 1.18 Schematic diagram of the utricular macula, demonstrating the effect of bending forward.

Ampullae of the semicircular canals The ampullae of the semicircular canals detect angular acceleration, for example the movement experienced on a merry-go-round (**Figure 1.19**). The ampulla contains the saddle-shaped crista, on which the hair cells sit. The stereocilia of the hair cells protrude into a gelatinous material called the cupula. With a turn of the head, the inertia of the endolymph in the semicircular canal causes the cupula to move, deflecting the stereocilia and stimulating transduction. Each semicircular canal is paired with one in a parallel plane on the opposite side of the head. One gives an excitatory response and the other an inhibitory response in a given plane.

Vestibular reflexes The vestibular system is involved in two reflexes:
- The **vestibulo-ocular reflex** co-ordinates and stabilises eye movement with head movement, so that objects can remain in focus and in fixed view. The interneurons are between the vestibular nuclei and the oculomotor and abducens nuclei.
- The **vestibulospinal reflexes** co-ordinate head and body movement with posture. The interneurons are between

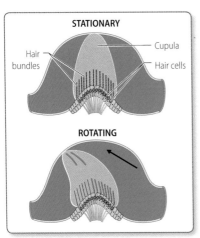

Figure 1.19 Schematic diagram of the ampulla of the lateral semicircular canal, demonstrating the effect of rotation.

Clinical insight

When the head is rotated to the right, the eyes move to the left in proportion to the stimulation, but are returned to the mid-position through a central corrective reflex. In clinical practice this is the basis for *nystagmus*, an involuntary movement of the eyes with a slow vestibular component followed by a faster central corrective component.

the vestibular nuclei and the vestibulospinal tract of the spinal cord, where they synapse with efferents to neck and posture muscles.

Physiology of smell

The olfactory system (**Figure 1.20**) allows distinction between large numbers of different smells.

Olfactory cells The olfactory area is a region of specialised sensory epithelium in the roof of the nasal cavity, with a surface area of 200–400 mm^2. Its surface area is further increased by the

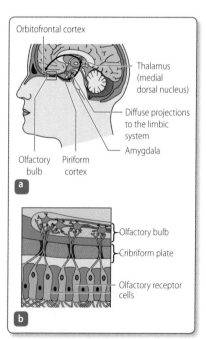

Figure 1.20 The olfactory system; (a) central pathways, (b) olfactory bulb detail.

Orbitofrontal cortex

Thalamus (medial dorsal nucleus)

Diffuse projections to the limbic system

Amygdala

Olfactory bulb

Piriform cortex

a

Olfactory bulb

Cribriform plate

Olfactory receptor cells

b

presence of receptor cells which have modified cilia and project into the mucus lining the nasal epithelium. Other types of cells of the olfactory epithelium include columnar supporting cells and basal cells. The basal cells continually divide to produce new olfactory receptor cells which, because of their short lifespan, need to be continually replaced. This is an unusual characteristic, because most other nerve cells cannot be regenerated.

Olfactory processes The process of sniffing ensures maximum exposure of odours to the olfactory area, via turbulent airflow. Odours that reach this area are absorbed into the water fraction of the mucus and in turn react with the lipid bilayer of the receptor cells at specific sites. This causes K^+ and Cl^- to flow out leading to depolarisation of the sensory cells. A slow *compound action potential* (i.e. the sum action potential of the multiple primary afferents) is generated from the olfactory mucosa. Depending on the chemical nature of the stimulus, the threshold varies: the threshold for perceiving a smell is lower than that required to identify a smell. There is also marked adaptation of the olfactory response, with an increase in threshold following exposure, but recovery occurs quickly.

Olfactory pathway

Each receptor cell is connected by non-myelinated nerve fibres to the olfactory glomeruli of the **olfactory bulb**. Each glomerulus receives about 25 000 fibres and fires in an 'all-or-nothing' fashion into the **mitral** or **tufted cells** of the olfactory bulb. These bulbar cells have (approximately 100 000 axons projecting along the olfactory tract (as the **olfactory nerve** (CN I)) to synapse at five cerebral regions:
- the piriform cortex
- the periamygdaloid area
- the olfactory tubercle
- the amygdala
- the entorhinal cortex.

Unlike other sensory pathways to the cerebral cortex, the olfactory pathway does not relay to the thalamus. However,

Clinical insight

Pathologies of taste

- *Hypogeusia* is reduced taste activity, whereas a total loss of taste is known as *ageusia*
- Saliva is necessary for taste perception, and abnormalities in its production (e.g. Sjögren's disease), or reduced saliva flow due to surgical removal of salivary glands or after radiotherapy, can lead to taste disturbance
- Other processes that can affect taste include vitamin A and B12 or zinc deficiencies, hypothyroidism, Cushing's disease, and various drugs including amitriptyline and cytotoxic agents.

fibres do leave the olfactory cortical areas and relay in the thalamus on their way to the hypothalamus or other areas, where they perhaps play a role in the regulation of the intake of food and other behaviours that depend on olfactory information.

Physiology of taste

The five primary taste submodalities are sweet, sour, salty, bitter and umami. The tip of the tongue is the most sensitive to sweetness and saltiness. The lateral aspects of the tongue are most sensitive to sourness, and the back of the tongue is most sensitive to bitterness. Umami is sensed throughout.

The taste buds are situated predominantly on raised tongue protrusions called **papillae** (**Figure 1.21**), of which there are four types:

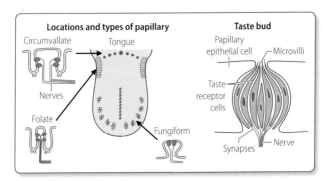

Figure 1.21 The tongue contains outward protrusions called papillae, of which there are three main types. Taste buds are situated in various locations on the papillae.

- **Fungiform papillae** at the anterior tip and sides of the tongue are 'mushroom-shaped'
- **Foliate papillae** are found at the base of the tongue
- **Circumvallate papillae** at the back of the tongue are in close proximity to gustatory gland ducts and are shaped to collect the lipase-containing secretions; there are usually only 10–14 in total
- **Filiform papillae** are long keratinised papillae that don't have taste buds.

There are also taste buds on the palate and lips. Taste buds are a collection of 50 to 100 elongated epithelial cells called **taste receptor cells** (TRCs) embedded in the papillar epithelium. They are of epithelial origin and undergo constant renewal. There are three types of cells in taste buds:

- Type I TRCs have tall microvilli and are thought to be support cells (i.e. glial-like)
- Type II TRCs have short microvilli and sense sweet, bitter and umami tastes
- Type III TRCs have a single thick microvillus and synapse with the adjacent gustatory nerve.

From each cell type, processes extend up into the pore region of the bud, and nerves enter and leave the taste bud through its base.

Physiology of voice

Voice production requires:

- An air source (the lungs)
- A vibratory source (the vocal folds)
- A resonating chamber (the pharynx, oral cavity and nose).

Any disorder of these components can contribute to changes in the voice.

Phonation   In order to phonate, the recurrent laryngeal nerves set the vocal folds into the adducted position. However, as the vocal processes of the arytenoid cartilages (forming the posterior one third) are more bulky than the membranous vocal folds, a slight gap exists between the vocal folds. The lungs then expel air, and this airstream passes through the gap. According to the Bernoulli principle, there is a drop in pressure at the site of the glottis and this causes the mucosa of the vocal folds to be drawn into the gap and block it. Subsequently, the sub-glottic pressure rises and causes another stream of air to pass through the glottis, followed again by a drop in pressure and glottic closure. Repeated cycles of this process set up a vibratory pattern in the vocal folds, and the resulting sound is what we interpret as voice. As the sound passes through the resonating chamber of the pharynx and oral cavity containing the palate, tongue, teeth and lips, this voice is further modulated into speech.

Guiding principle

The Bernoulli principle

- States that for constant flow of a fluid or gas, as the velocity increases the pressure decreases
- Therefore, when air passes from the lungs to the pharynx through the constriction of the glottis, the velocity is greatest and the pressure least at the site of constriction.

Pitch The tension and length of the vocal folds together with the tracheal air pressure are important in determining the pitch of the voice. Vocal fold length is altered by the cricothyroid and thyroarytenoid muscles. Shortening of the vocal folds leads to the tension being readjusted by the vocalis muscle. An increase in tension with maintenance of vocal fold length, as with raising the voice, leads to a rise in pitch. An increase in volume is attained by a rise of air pressure associated with a reduction in the elasticity of the glottis.

Physiology of swallowing

Swallowing is the mechanism that transmits liquids or solids from the mouth to the stomach, via the pharynx and oesophagus, without entering the respiratory tract. Although it is initiated voluntarily there are involuntary components, with complex neuromuscular involvement. Swallowing has three stages (**Figure 1.22**):

- oral
- pharyngeal
- oesophageal.

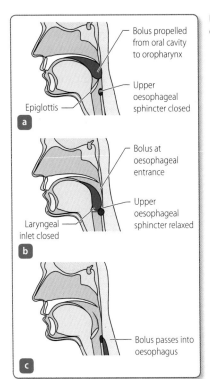

Figure 1.22 The stages of swallowing.

Labels in figure:
- Bolus propelled from oral cavity to oropharynx
- Upper oesophageal sphincter closed
- Epiglottis
- a
- Bolus at oesophageal entrance
- Upper oesophageal sphincter relaxed
- Laryngeal inlet closed
- b
- Bolus passes into oesophagus
- c

Oral stage

This begins when fluid or food is placed into the mouth. As well as closure of the lips it requires closure of the oropharyngeal sphincter so that material is retained in the mouth until ready to progress into the pharynx. Solids require preparation to form a bolus, with co-ordinated action from the lips and buccal, mandibular and tongue movements for chewing to break up the particles and mix them with saliva. The cranial nerves involved are:

- the trigeminal nerve (sensation and mastication)
- the facial nerve (lips and buccal movements)
- the vagus nerve (oropharyngeal sphincter)
- the hypoglossal nerve (tongue movements).

The bolus is assembled between the tongue and the hard palate. Contraction of the tongue in co-ordinated fashion from front to back propels the bolus posteriorly into the oropharynx with relaxation of the palatoglossal sphincter. The soft palate is pulled posterosuperiorly to close the nasopharynx to stop respiration and prevent nasal regurgitation.

Pharyngeal stage

The pharyngeal stage is completed within 1 second and involves the tongue base acting as a piston, pumping the bolus towards the entrance of the oesophagus, as well as the elevation of the larynx by the suprahyoid muscles. This gives rise to a negative pressure in the entrance of the oesophagus. There is associated relaxation of the upper oesophageal sphincter, allowing the bolus into the oesophagus. Movement of the leading edge of the bolus into the oesophagus triggers the pharyngeal constrictor muscles to contract from above downwards, propelling the bolus into the oesophagus. During this phase both the laryngeal inlet and the nasopharynx are closed to prevent aspiration and nasal regurgitation. The sensory input travels via the glossopharyngeal and vagus nerves.

Oesophageal stage

The oesophageal stage lasts 8–20 seconds; it begins with the bolus entering the oesophagus and ends when it has passed through the lower oesophageal sphincter into the stomach. Peristaltic waves can be primary, passing down the oesophagus, or secondary arising locally in response to distension of the oesophagus, helping transport the bolus through the oesophagus. Tertiary oesophageal contractions are irregular and non-propulsive, involving long segments of the oesophagus and frequently developing during emotional stress. The lower oesophageal sphincter is regulated by the vagus nerve.

Clinical essentials

2.1 Introduction

In this chapter history taking and examination are subdivided into regions for convenience, whereas in reality the ear, nose and throat are interrelated and the pathology of one region can present with symptoms of another; alternatively, the cause may be at a distant location. For example, nasopharyngeal swelling can present with hearing loss, or lung tumour may present with hoarseness secondary to recurrent laryngeal nerve involvement.

2.2 History taking

A systematic approach to history taking is relevant to all medical specialties, and the ear, nose and throat are no exception.

Otology

The cardinal symptoms of ear disease are otalgia, discharge, hearing loss, tinnitus, vertigo, and aural fullness (**Table 2.1**).

Otalgia (ear pain)

Common causes of ear pain include:

- Otitis media, the most common cause of otalgia. A throbbing pain which resolves suddenly may indicate spontaneous perforation of the tympanic membrane with release of the pus from the middle ear into the ear canal
- Earache due to barotrauma during flights, when the outer and middle ear pressure fails to equalise
- Severe otitis externa (infection of the outer ear). This can be excruciatingly painful as the skin of the external meatus is particularly sensitive
- Local trauma

Rare causes of ear pain include:

- Herpes zoster oticus, even before vesicles are seen

Presenting symptom	Common causes
Hearing loss	**Sensorineural** – noise-induced hearing loss, presbyacusis, ototoxicity, acoustic neuroma, systemic causes, congenital causes, temporal bone trauma **Conductive** – wax impaction, otitis media (acute), otitis media with effusion, middle ear and ossicular pathology, chronic suppurative otitis media, Eustachian tube dysfunction and blockage, otosclerosis, barotrauma
Vertigo	Ménière's disease, benign paroxysmal positional vertigo, vestibular neuronitis, labyrinthitis, perilymph fistula
Otorrhoea	Otitis externa, acute otitis media with perforation, chronic suppurative otitis media, malignant otitis externa, leakage of cerebrospinal fluid
Otalgia	Otitis media, otitis externa, trauma, herpes zoster oticus, polychondritis helicis, myringitis bullosa haemorrhagica
Facial asymmetry	Bell's (idiopathic) palsy, herpes zoster oticus, trauma, 'malignant' (necrotising) otitis externa
Tinnitus	Ménière's disease, noise-induced hearing loss, presbyacusis, ototoxicity, acoustic neuroma, temporal bone trauma, perilymph fistula

Table 2.1 Presenting ear symptoms and common causes/likely diagnosis

- Referred otalgia from pathology in the areas supplied by cervical nerves or cranial nerves V, VII, IX and X, i.e. neck, oral cavity, sinuses, pharynx, larynx and dental problems
- Malignancy, e.g. squamous cell carcinoma.

Discharge

The type of discharge may give a clear indication as to the site of pathology.

- If mucus is present the discharge originates from the middle ear cleft, as the skin of the external canal has no mucous glands

- Clear fluid discharge following head injury suggests a CSF leak from a skull base fracture (usually middle cranial fossa). A thick brown discharge is usually liquefied wax
- A foul-smelling scanty discharge, often greenish-yellow with keratinous debris, is a hallmark of cholesteatoma
- Serosanguineous discharge is associated with granulations and rarely neoplastic lesions. Fresh bleeding is common after trauma, and less commonly, due to vascular tumours
- In chronic otitis media the discharge is usually long standing, with acute exacerbations.

Hearing loss

It is important to establish the nature of the onset of hearing loss (sudden or gradually progressive), the type (stable or fluctuating, unilateral or bilateral) and whether it is associated with any other otological symptoms, such as tinnitus, vertigo, discharge or otalgia. Sensorineural hearing loss results from cochlear and retrocochlear pathology, which reduces speech discrimination. Conductive hearing loss is mainly due to pathology of the middle ear and the external auditory canal (EAC).

> **Guiding principle**
>
> A thorough general history should carefully document:
> - systemic illnesses
> - medication with any potential ototoxic drugs (e.g. aminoglycosides, loop diuretics or salicylates)
> - family history (otosclerosis)
> - occupational and social history (exposure to loud noise, recent trauma or otological surgery)

Tinnitus

The type of tinnitus is a useful pointer:
- **pulsatile tinnitus** is suggestive of a vascular lesion
- **dull, lower frequency, continuous tinnitus** could coexist with a conductive loss due to a reduction in the level of background noise getting through the middle ear
- **high-frequency hissing and ringing** is commonly seen with sensorineural hearing loss due to cochlear or neural pathology

- **fluctuant tinnitus** (along with episodic vertigo and hearing loss) is a feature of endolymphatic hydrops (Ménière's disease) or, rarely, perilymph fistula.

Vertigo

Vertigo is an illusion of movement (rotatory or horizontal) and must be distinguished from disequilibrium (usually a central cause), syncope (usually a cardiac cause) and light-headedness (panic attacks or hyperventilation).

History taking is of paramount importance in vertigo, as diagnosis of the cause is often made by history alone. The first attack needs to be described in detail. Specific questions can establish the likely diagnosis and should explore:

- **onset**, whether sudden or gradual
- **precipitating or exacerbating factors** (e.g. positional change in benign paroxysmal positional vertigo)
- **duration** (seconds, minutes, hours or days)
- **associated symptoms** (nausea, vomiting, hearing loss, tinnitus or neurological symptoms)
- **nature**, whether episodic (Ménière's disease) or constant.

Aural fullness and facial weakness

These can present as symptoms of ear disease; they are usually non-specific and associated with other otological symptoms. **Facial asymmetry** is associated with the facial nerve being affected in its course through the temporal bone. **Facial nerve paralysis** is seen in Bell's palsy (idiopathic), in Ramsay Hunt syndrome (herpes zoster), in trauma, and rarely with tumours or severe infections involving the skull base and temporal bone.

Clinical insight

Acute sinus pathology can also result in **eye symptoms** (e.g. double vision or protrusion of the eye) and can affect visual acuity and/or loss of colour vision.

Rhinology

Patients with nasal and sinus pathology present with nasal blockage, rhinorrhoea, postnasal drip, nasal congestion and crusting, loss or diminution of sensation of smell and taste, nasal bleeding (epistaxis) and headaches, usually frontoethmoidal. Nasal itching and sneezing usually have an allergic cause, and facial pain is unlikely to be sinugenic in origin unless there is an active infection where there is pain over the cheek (maxillary sinusitis) or orbit and forehead (frontal sinusitis).

Nasal obstruction

Unless proved otherwise, unilateral nasal obstruction in a child is usually due to a foreign body. A gradually progressing obstruction could be due to slowly growing nasal polyps. It is common with the nasal cycle for one side of the nose to be blocked, and generally the side alternates during the day. If the blockage is constant on one side there is likely to be a structural lesion, such as a deviated septum. A unilateral blockage that is worsening and associated with bleeding needs urgent assessment to rule out a tumour.

Rhinorrhoea

Rhinorrhoea is nasal discharge. The type of nasal discharge indicates the aetiology:

- Allergic rhinitis is commonly associated with clear, watery rhinorrhoea
- Rarely, clear fluid is due to spontaneous or post-traumatic CSF rhinorrhoea
- Mucoid or mucopurulent discharge is commonly seen in infective and chronic rhinosinusitis.

A nasal discharge can be anterior or postnasal, often termed postnasal drip. This could result in episodes of throat clearing secondary to laryngeal and pharyngeal irritation, which can often turn into habitual throat clearing.

Epistaxis

Epistaxis (bleeding from the nose) and bloodstained discharge can be due to a variety of causes – as trivial as a result of nose-picking in children and young adults, to local infective causes, and systemic disorders affecting coagulation. It's important to take a medication history to elicit use of drugs such as aspirin or warfarin that affect coagulation. Nasal bleeds could also be indicative of chronic granulomatous conditions and more sinister pathology such as tumours.

Alteration of sense of smell

This can be a result of blockage of the olfactory receptors by mucus or polyps, or damage to the olfactory pathway by frontal trauma.

Head and neck

The cardinal features of history relevant to head and neck pathology include sore throat, hoarseness or change in voice (dysphonia), the presence of a lump in the neck, feeling of a lump in the throat (globus pharyngeus), heartburn due to acid reflux, snoring, noisy breathing (stridor or stertor, depending on the site of origin of the noise), and difficulty swallowing (dysphagia). Cough, referred earache, throat clearing, halitosis and a foul taste in the mouth could be due to conditions in the head and neck or adjoining regions.

Sore throat

This is the most common presenting symptom and ranges from mild, due to common viral infections of the upper respiratory tract affecting the pharynx, to severe in bacterial tonsillitis or quite severe in quinsy (a collection of pus lateral to the tonsil).

Hoarseness or change in voice

Hoarseness is often due to a pathology affecting the vocal cord or its neural pathways. Remember that the recurrent laryngeal nerve, which supplies the majority of the laryngeal muscles, can be affected in the chest (e.g. by lung cancer or mediastinal node pathology) or may be traumatised in thyroid or cardiac surgery. Prolonged or overuse of the voice is seen in occupations such as teaching and singing.

Globus pharyngeus

This is a feeling of a lump in the throat without true dysphagia to solids or liquids. It is usually intermittent, is often felt at the region of the sternal notch or higher, and can be unilateral. It is often associated with anxiety and stress, although it can be a manifestation of reflux oesophagitis and disorders of pharyngo-oesopharyngeal motility, e.g. cricopharyngeal muscle spasms.

Dysphagia

Dysphagia is difficulty in swallowing. True dysphagia is usually constant, and one must consider any physical cause for the symptom, such as a postcricoid carcinoma, foreign body or pharyngeal pouch. Patients require further investigations, including barium swallow or endoscopic assessment.

Acid reflux and heartburn

Besides suggesting gastro-oesophageal reflux disease, acid reflux and heartburn account for many laryngeal symptoms resulting from posterior laryngitis (excess acid exposure around the back of the throat and larynx – termed laryngopharyngeal reflux). Hoarseness, dry cough, constant throat clearing and a foul taste in the mouth are common presenting symptoms of reflux disease.

Halitosis

Halitosis (bad breath) commonly results from a coated tongue. Other causes include pathology of the mouth and gums, nose and sinuses, stomach and oesophagus, as well as tonsiloliths and systemic disease.

Swelling of the neck

Neck lumps commonly present in the ENT clinic. The swelling can be caused by pathology at the site of the lump (e.g. a multinodular goitre, submandibular sialadenitis or branchial cyst) or it can be the result of pathology at a distant site (e.g. swelling of jugulodigastric lymph nodes from recurrent tonsillitis or lymph node tumours secondary to a primary neoplastic lesion in the oropharynx). The origin, duration, progress, size, site or location often indicates the nature of the swelling – this is dealt with in detail in other chapters.

Snoring

This common cause of marital disharmony can be due to palatal flutter or pharyngeal or nasal causes. In all cases a history of sleep apnoea should be sought, as snoring can be part of the obstructive sleep apnoea syndrome, which is associated with a much higher morbidity than simple snoring without apnoea.

Stridor and stertor

Stridor is a high-pitched noise caused by partial obstruction of the respiratory tract at or below the larynx. It needs to be differentiated from stertor, a lower-pitched inspiratory snoring sound resulting from obstructions above the level of the larynx. Depending on the severity of the symptoms, both of these presentations need urgent assessment by the otolaryngologist, particularly in children.

Special considerations in the child

In children the history often comes not from the child but from the parent, guardian or carer. The doctor often has to deal with both an anxious child and an even more anxious parent.

Congenital conditions

The majority of congenital conditions manifest in the early years, and the perinatal history is important in identifying risk factors for both acquired and congenital conditions.

Congenital hearing loss is now picked up early at newborn screening; in the younger child speech and language delay could be an early indicator of hearing deficit, and behavioural issues, head shaking and to some extent balance problems could point towards ear conditions where a full paediatric audiological assessment is indicated.

Epistaxis in a child is common and the vast majority respond to topical medication. Unilateral nasal discharge in a child, unless proved otherwise, is usually due to a foreign body, but a history of insertion of the foreign body may not be forthcoming! Choanal atresia, if bilateral, presents in newborns as cyanotic spells relieved by crying, as children are obligate nose breathers. Unilateral atresia may present later in childhood.

Airways

The airways in the child are narrower and more tenuous than in adults. In any child with a history of respiratory distress (cyanosis, apnoea, dyspnoea, stridor) the potential for airway emergencies is high. Laryngomalacia, the most common cause of stridor in children, is self-limiting in 90% and symptoms regress as the child grows. For most other conditions the child must be assessed by a paediatric otolaryngologist.

2.3 Clinical examination

It is good medical practice and reassuring for the patient to use antibacterial hand rub before and *after* the examination, and to use a new speculum for each side of the ear or nose if you are using the auriscope. Adequate illumination and exposure are essential. Always ask about tenderness and establish which is the affected side – it is better to examine the 'good' side first and the affected side next. The ENT instruments commonly used for clinical examination are shown in **Figure 2.1**.

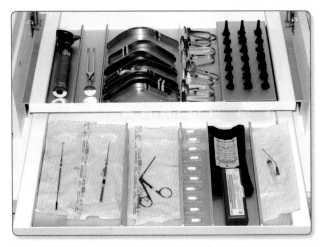

Figure 2.1 ENT instrument tray. Upper level (from left to right): otoscope, tuning fork, Lacs tongue depressor, Thudicum's nasal specula, ear specula. Lower level (from left to right): Jobson Horne probe, ear (wax) hook, aural forceps, ear wicks, silver nitrate cautery, local anaesthetic spray, syringe and cannula for instillation of aural medication.

Ear

Clinical examination of the ear begins from the outside (pinna, preaural and postaural regions) and proceeds systematically inside the external auditory canal (EAC) to the tympanic membrane, repeating for the other side.

Adequate illumination with an otoscope (auriscope) is essential, particularly to observe the colour of the tympanic membrane. The pre- and postaural regions are inspected for scars (easily missed) or sinuses. The pinna is inspected and gently pulled backwards and upwards (in an older child or adult) or backwards and downwards (in infants) to straighten the external meatus. Choose the largest speculum that can be inserted easily and attach this to the otoscope. Pneumatic otoscopes have an attachment to check the mobility of the tympanic membrane.

The otoscope with the speculum is gently inserted into the meatus, holding the pinna as in **Figure 2.2**. The EAC is inspected for any wax or debris or obvious pathology, including the bony outgrowths seen in benign osteomas (**Figure 2.3**) or surfer's and

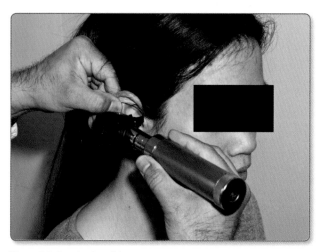

Figure 2.2 Examination of the ear using an otoscope.

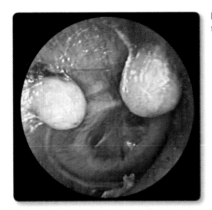

Figure 2.3 Osteoma of the ear canal.

swimmer's exostoses. The speculum is gently inserted further and all four quadrants of the tympanic membrane are inspected by varying the angle of the speculum.

The normal tympanic membrane is translucent white with the characteristic cone of light (see **Figure 1.4**). Carefully inspect the attic (pars flaccida) for any pits, debris or keratin. Make a note of any pathology including scarring, chalky white features of tympanosclerosis, keratin debris suggestive of cholesteatoma, retraction, and dull appearance of the tympanic membrane or any fluid levels or bubbles behind it. If there is a perforation (**Figure 2.4**) note its site, size and margins (or lack of); occasionally middle ear structures can be visualised through the perforation. A postaural or endaural scar is probably a result of surgery; in these cases look particularly for features of mastoid surgery, for example a mastoid cavity, where part of the posterior superior wall of the acoustic meatus may be missing.

Clinical assessment of deafness

Clinical assessment of hearing is useful to determine the type and degree of deafness.

- Conductive deafness is usually correctable by surgery and commonly results from pathology in the outer or middle ear.

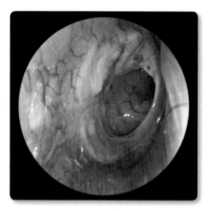

Figure 2.4 Perforation of the right tympanic membrane, with an area of tympanosclerosis in the posterior superior quadrant.

The sound waves are prevented from reaching the cochlea by a failure of the coupling or transformer mechanisms involving the outer or middle ear

- Sensorineural deafness results from abnormal or defective function or absence of the cochlear neuroepithelium or the auditory nerve. The neural impulses are prevented from reaching the auditory cortex of the brain
- Mixed deafness results from a combination of conductive and sensorineural deafness in varying proportions affecting the same ear.

The first assessment of hearing in the history-taking is by observing how well the patient hears and responds, and should be monitored throughout the consultation. Audiograms can be misleading, and it is always more clinically useful to correlate voice, whisper and tuning fork tests to the audiometry findings.

Formal assessment with free field speech testing is made by asking the patient to repeat bisyllabic words or numbers. The examiner will need to mask the non-test ear by either gently occluding the EAC or rubbing the tragus of the other ear; if profound unilateral deafness is suspected then a Barany noise box is used to mask the 'good' ear.

The results are recorded with a whispered voice and a conversational voice at varying distances from the ear (e.g. 6 inches, 2 feet).

Tuning fork tests

The tuning fork used for tests is 512 Hz (frequency in cycles per second), which is a frequency common in human speech. There are two tuning fork tests, Rinne's and Weber's, which complement each other.

Rinne's test

This is a test of middle ear function. It relies on the fact that the conduction of sound through the EAC, ('air conduction', 'AC') is better than conduction of sound through the mastoid bone ('bone conduction', 'BC'), because the middle ear transformer mechanism (see page 24) increases the sound energy transmitted to the cochlea to a greater extent than would occur from a direct coupling.

The tuning fork is struck and the prongs are held close to the EAC, testing air conduction, and then its base is placed firmly on the mastoid process, testing bone conduction. The sound intensities are then compared:

- **If air conduction is greater** (i.e. louder) than bone conduction, the middle and outer ears are functioning normally and the test is Rinne positive: AC>BC. This could occur in a normal ear or with sensorineural deafness.
- **If bone conduction is greater** (louder) than air conduction, the middle and outer ears are not functioning normally and the test is Rinne negative: BC>AC. This denotes conductive deafness.

Rinne's test can be falsely negative if there is profound sensorineural deafness (see page 51 and **Figure 2.6**).

Weber test

This test is useful in determining the type of deafness and comparing the cochlear function of the two ears. The tuning fork is struck and held in the middle of the skull equidistant from the two ears; other midline sites sometimes used are the front of the forehead, the chin or the teeth. The patient is asked whether the sound is heard equally on both sides (centrally), or louder or referred to one ear (lateralised to one ear).

- **In normal hearing**, the sound is heard centrally or equally loud in both ears (no lateralisation) (**Figure 2.5a**). A patient with symmetrical hearing loss will also hear the sound equally, so the test is useful only in asymmetrical hearing loss
- **In sensorineural loss**, the sound is heard louder or is lateralised to the 'better' ear, as the better-functioning cochlea hears the sound louder (**Figure 2.5b**)

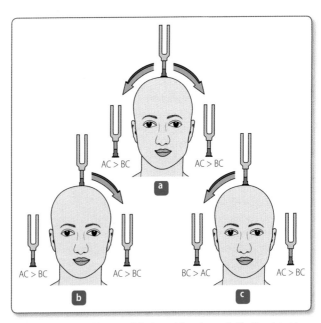

Figure 2.5 (a) Normal hearing. Weber's test is heard centrally. The Rinne's test is positive on both sides, with air conduction greater than bone conduction. (b) Sensorineural deafness in the right ear: Weber's test lateralises to the better-hearing (left) side. Rinne's test is positive on both sides. (c) Conductive deafness in the right ear. Weber's test lateralises to the affected right ear. Rinne's test is negative on the right side (BC > AC) and positive on the normal left side (AC > BC).

- **In unilateral conductive hearing loss**, the sound is perceived as being louder in the affected ear. This is because the conductive loss masks the ambient noise of the room, and the cochlea more easily picks up the presented sound via the bones of the skull, causing it to be perceived as louder than in the unaffected ear (**Figure 2.5c**).

Clinical insight

Beware of the false-negative Rinne test: a negative Rinne's test can be falsely interpreted as conductive hearing loss in the presence of *profound* sensorineural deafness. This can only be confirmed after the Weber test is performed. In contrast to conductive hearing loss, in the presence of profound deafness the Weber test lateralises to the opposite normal ear. An example of the false-negative Rinne's test is shown diagrammatically in **Figure 2.6**.

Facial nerve assessment

This is an essential part of clinical examination of the ear. The motor functions of the facial nerve muscles are tested by lifting the forehead, raising the eyebrows, screwing the eyes tightly (test strength), puffing or blowing of the cheeks, and showing the teeth and smiling.

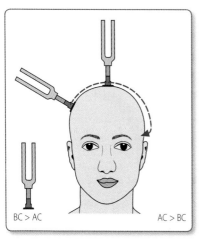

BC > AC   AC > BC

Figure 2.6 Although Rinne's test is apparently negative (BC >AC) on the right side, it can be seen that the sound (BC) is travelling transcranially from the right mastoid to the normal left cochlea.

Fistula test and pneumatic otoscopy

Movement of the tympanic membrane can be seen using a Siegle speculum (**Figure 2.7**). If there is scarring of the membrane or fluid behind it, movement is impaired. The fistula test is carried out by applying intermittent firm pressure over the tragus for a few seconds; watch for deviation of the eyes away from the examined side and then nystagmus (jerky eye movements) in the direction of the diseased side; if positive, this could suggest a communication between the middle and the inner ear, e.g. perilymphatic leak or fistula.

Nose

Clinical examination of the nose requires adequate illumination, either reflected by a head mirror from a bulls-eye lamp or directly from a head lamp or otoscope, or with a rigid endoscope. Before examining the inside of the nose inspect the external nose from the front, from the side and from below. Nasal humps and depressions are better seen from the side. Gently lift the tip of the nose to look for any deviation or anterior caudal dislocation of the septum.

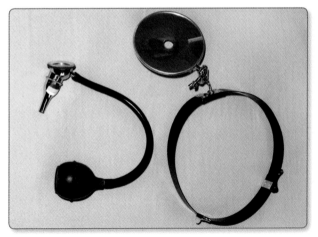

Figure 2.7 A Siegle speculum for pneumatic otoscopy; head mirror.

Assessment

The assessment of airways and patency can start even before a nasal speculum is introduced. Hold a cool polished metal surface (e.g. the flat end of a metal tongue depressor) below the nostrils and ask the patient to breathe out gently while occluding one nostril at a time (**Figure 2.8**). Compare the area of 'misting' or condensation on each side: a reduced area of misting on one side denotes obstruction on that side.

Interior of the nose

The interior of the nose can be visualised using an otoscope and a speculum; sometimes lifting the nasal tip with the thumb provides an adequate view. In adults a Thudicum's speculum may be used, although the best illumination and magnification are provided by an endoscope. As the nasal cavity extends horizontally backwards by about 7 cm, the angle of approach is horizontal rather than upwards. The area best visualised with an endoscope is the middle meatal area, where the majority of the sinuses drain.

Nasal lining

The nasal lining and turbinates are sensitive to touch and are vascular. The polypoidal inferior turbinate can be easily confused with a nasal polyp; however, a polyp is usually greyish,

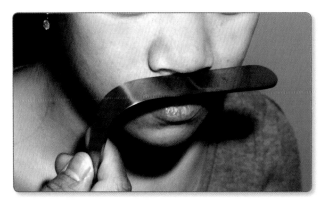

Figure 2.8 Examining the patency of the nasal airways by observing condensation on a metal surface.

insensate and not as vascular. A decongestant spray will shrink a vascular polypoidal turbinate but not a polyp.

Throat

The oral cavity and pharynx are inspected with good illumination using a tongue depressor. The tonsils, faucial pillars, soft and hard palate and posterior pharyngeal wall are inspected; two depressors are used to inspect the buccal mucosa, the gums on both sides and the openings of the parotid duct. The under-surface of the tongue, the floor of the mouth and the openings of the submandibular glands on either side of the frenulum are inspected. Complete the examination by bimanual palpation with a gloved finger in the oral cavity, palpating the base of the tongue for any swelling and the submandibular glands and duct for stones.

Indirect laryngoscopy

In indirect laryngoscopy the tongue is stabilised with the thumb and the middle finger and a warmed laryngeal mirror introduced firmly against the soft palate; the laryngeal structures are visualised by tilting the mirror. The patient is asked to phonate to say 'eee', which adducts the vocal folds (they move to the midline), and then to breathe deeply to abduct the vocal folds (they move away from the midline).

Fibreoptic endoscopy

Indirect laryngoscopy has largely been replaced by endoscopic assessment, where the findings can be documented and recorded simultaneously by attaching a camera to the endoscope. Rigid and flexible fibreoptic nasendoscopes are used to visualise the nasopharynx and to look for any pathologies in the postnasal space. The flexible nasendoscope is then introduced further to examine the hypopharyngeal region and larynx, including vocal folds, subglottis and upper tracheal rings, through the open (abducted) vocal folds (**Figure 2.9**).

Head and neck

Head and neck examination is best carried out in a systematic fashion with good illumination, proper positioning and

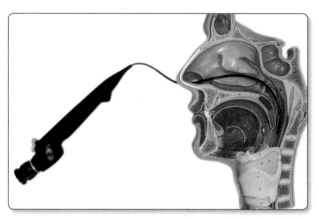

Figure 2.9 A flexible laryngoscope with a fibre optic light source is used to examine the nasal cavity, nasopharynx, hypopharynx and larynx.

adequate exposure of the neck to the level of the clavicles. Inspect the neck for any scars, sinuses, skin changes and swellings. For obvious visible swellings ask the patient to take a sip of water, hold it in their mouth and then swallow, to assess movement. Any swelling attached to the pretracheal fascia (e.g. the thyroid) moves with swallowing. For midline swellings ask the patient to protrude their tongue; a thyroglossal cyst moves with tongue protrusion.

Check with the patient that there is no tenderness before approaching to palpate the neck from the back. Position the head and neck in neutral and define the lower border of the mandible (**Figure 2.10a**). Move systematically from the submental, submandibular and parotid regions to the anterior border of the sternocleidomastoid and complete palpation of the lymph node chains in the anterior neck. Do not forget the posterior triangle. Palpate the supraclavicular region, moving upwards along the posterior border of sternocleidomastoid. Move up the midline to include the trachea, thyroid and larynx (**Figure 2.10b**). Laryngeal crepitus or 'crackling' is normally felt on moving the larynx from side to side.

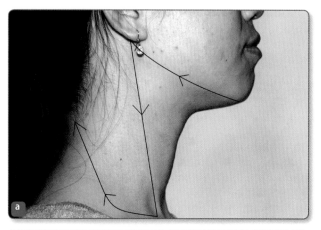

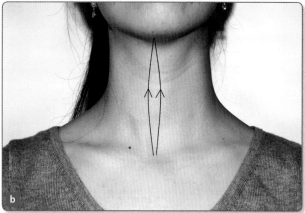

Figure 2.10 Examination of the neck is carried out systematically in the direction of the arrows.

Lumps in the neck

Any lump in the neck should be noted for size, consistency, fluctuance, mobility, tethering to underlying or overlying structures, level (see **Figure 1.11,** page 15), pulsatility, borders, tenderness, presence of a punctum, and transillumination (if the swelling is cystic). Listen for a bruit (if the swelling is likely to be vascular). Percussion is useful for determining retrosternal extension of a large goitre.

Thyroid status

Thyroid status is also determined by examining the hands and eyes. The hands are looked at carefully for tremors and skin texture (look for palmar erythema and vitiligo), the fingers for onycholysis and clubbing. The hands are felt for sweatiness, and the rate and rhythm of the pulse noted. The face and eyes are examined for exophthalmos, proptosis, lid lag, lid retraction, chemosis and ophthalmoplegia. Look also for pretibial myxoedema and check deep tendon reflexes.

Neurological examination

Relevant neurological assessment, which involves testing the cranial nerves, is described in **Table 2.2**.

The corneal reflex is dependent on the integrity of the Vth and the VIIth cranial nerves. The method for testing the corneal reflex is given in **Table 2.3**.

2.4 Investigations

Although a proper history and examination are essential for formulating a differential diagnosis, specific investigations are sometimes required for a definitive diagnosis. This section aims to create an awareness of the commonly used investigations in otolaryngology, although the choice of specific investigation will be discussed under each topic chapter. In general, investigations can be grouped under the type of investigative technique:

- haematological (blood tests)
- microbiological
- radiological (including nuclear medicine)
- histocytopathological
- audiological.

Cranial nerve(s)	Assessment
Optic [I] and oculomotor [III]	Look for ptosis (weakness of levator palpebrae superioris due to third nerve palsy or tarsal muscle weakness due to Horner's syndrome) Pupil size: test accommodation (distant and 12 cm from nasal bridge fixation) and light reflex (swinging torch) Check eye movements Test acuity using Snellen charts and visual fields with perimetry
Trigeminal [V]	Test all three sensory divisions and corneal reflex (see **Table 2.3**). Also test strength of muscles of mastication (motor)
Facial [VII]	Ask the patient to raise eyebrows, screw eyes shut (test strength), wrinkle nose, blow out cheeks (test strength), show teeth
Glossopharyngeal [IX], vagus [X], hypoglossal [XII]	Tell the patient: 'Open your mouth, say "ahhh"' Check palatal movement and sound of 'ahh' Observe tongue for fasciculations Ask patient to point the tongue to the left, and then to the right
Accessory [X]	Tell the patient to turn his/her head to the right/left and push your hands away with his/her chin Tell the patient 'Shrug your shoulders'
Cerebellum	Past-pointing: 'With your index finger, touch my finger…now touch your nose…and keep going back and forth' Test for dysdiadochokinesis (inability to perform rapidly alternating movements) by asking the patient to rapidly pronate and supinate one hand on the other Heel-to-shin co-ordination
Gait	Romberg's test Heel-to-toe co-ordination with eyes open then closed Unterberger's stepping test Dix Hallpike manoeuvre for benign paroxysmal positional vertigo

Table 2.2 Cranial nerve assessment and neurological tests

Method	Distract the patient by asking him or her to gaze upwards Lightly touch the cornea with a wisp of cotton wool, approaching from the lateral side of the eye
Interpretation	*Normal:* reflex blinking of both eyes: *Facial nerve palsy:* patient can feel the touch of the cotton wool (via the ophthalmic division of the trigeminal nerve) but there is no reflex blink (via facial nerve innervation of orbicularis oris) *Trigeminal nerve palsy:* unable to feel touch of cotton wool

Table 2.3 Testing the corneal reflex

Haematological

A full blood count (FBC) and urea and electrolytes are generally considered 'routine' blood tests and often ignored, yet their results can help with both diagnosis and treatment. For example, in a patient presenting with an acute sore throat the white cell count (WBC) is usually moderately elevated, with a neutrophilia of around $12–25 \times 10^9$ per litre of blood in bacterial tonsillitis, whereas a markedly elevated level should make one suspicious of an acute leukaemia. Conversely, a low white cell count should prompt one to look for causes of leucopenia, which include immunodeficiency states. Urea and electrolytes not only guide one to the level of hydration and renal function, but can sometimes be useful in deriving a diagnosis in specific conditions such as secondary endolymphatic hydrops precipitated by an electrolyte imbalance. The blood tests that are most commonly used in ENT are listed in **Table 2.4**, although this is not an exhaustive list.

Microbiological

Microbiological tests are used to identify a causative pathogen as well as determine the correct choice of treatment, depending on drug sensitivities. Blood culture is used to identify the presence of systemic infection and the causative pathogen. Pus or fluid swabs from various sites, including the ear, nose and throat, can be sent for microbiological analysis. Fresh tissue

Test	Description
CRP	Marker of inflammation; useful in monitoring response to treatment
ACE	Elevated in 50–80% of patients with active sarcoidosis. Changes with disease activity
cANCA	Positive in 90% of patients with active Wegener's granulomatosis
RF	Elevated in connective tissue/autoimmune diseases (primarily used in diagnosis of RA and Sjögren's syndrome)
Anti-SS-A (Ro)	In Sjögren's syndrome, positive in ≤75%; may also be positive in SLE and scleroderma
Anti-SS-B (La)	In Sjögren's syndrome, positive in ≤60%; may also be positive in SLE and scleroderma; rarely present without anti-SS-A
ANA	Positive result suggests autoimmune disease, but specific tests are required for definitive diagnosis
Allergen-specific IgE antibody test	Tests allergy to common inhalant and food allergens; results are unaffected by oral antihistamines
Immunoglobulins (IgA, IgG, IgM)	Evaluates immune status of patients who present with recurrent infections
Autoantibody tests	Assist in diagnosing autoimmune disorders (NB individual tests are not diagnostic in isolation)
EBV antibodies	Positive result suggests current or very recent EBV infection
Thyroid function test, thyroid autoantibody	TSH evaluates thyroid activity and is useful in monitoring thyroid hormone replacement therapy. Thyroid autoantibody aids in diagnosis/monitoring of autoimmune thyroid diseases
Serological tests	Specific antibody tests for individual diseases, e.g. measles, mumps, rubella, HIV
QuantiFERON-TB Gold test (QFT)	Confirms *Mycobacterium tuberculosis* in latent and active disease

ACE, angiotensin-converting enzyme; ANA, antinuclear antibody test; cANCA, cytoplasmic antineutrophil cytoplasmic antibodies; CRP, C-reactive protein; EBV, Epstein–Barr virus; HIV, human immunodeficiency virus; Ig, immunoglobulin; RA, rheumatoid arthritis; RF, rheumatoid factor; SLE, systemic lupus erythematosus; TSH, thyroid-stimulating hormone.

Table 2.4 Blood tests commonly used in ENT

samples can be particularly useful when there is a suspicion of tuberculosis, or a fungal or unusual infection. An example would be a case of unresolving otitis externa, despite topical antibiotic and steroid eardrops, where a microbiology swab may reveal a fungal infection and aid correct topical antimicrobial treatment.

Radiological

Diagnostic imaging is essential for evaluating many otolaryngological conditions. Various modalities are available, including plain radiography with or without contrast, ultrasound, cross-sectional imaging (CT, MRI, PET) and nuclear medicine studies. As cross-sectional imaging has developed, plain radiography is less frequently employed. Plain sinus radiographs are rarely used as CT is superior, although they may be useful in acute sinusitis prior to considering a simple antral washout. CT of the temporal bones has replaced plain mastoid radiographs, although a modified Stenver's view may be useful in the postoperative assessment of a cochlear implant. Ultrasound has also taken precedence over plain radiographs for evaluating salivary gland calculi. However, plain soft-tissue lateral neck radiographs are still commonly used to evaluate foreign bodies in the throat.

Clinical insight

For the majority of common and uncomplicated infections (tonsillitis, otitis externa, otitis media and rhinosinusitis) it is not necessary to send microbiological samples and treatment can be commenced empirically. However, where there is failure to resolve with standard medical therapy it is prudent to send microbiological samples and discuss the case with the microbiologist. There may be local variations in antibiotic resistance, and ideally treatment should take this into consideration and be guided by the local hospital antibiotic policy.

Clinical insight

CT scanning is superior for bony detail, for example CT temporal bones for chronic middle ear disease, as well as CT paranasal sinuses for chronic rhinosinusitis.

MRI scanning is superior for soft tissue detail and exploits differences in tissue relaxation characteristics to produce an image which is very sensitive to contrast.

MRI with gadolinium contrast is especially useful in imaging tumours, such as acoustic neuromas, as well as in head and neck cancer.

Histological/cytopathological

In many cases an accurate diagnosis can only be obtained after a representative sample of the biopsied diseased tissue has been sent for microscopic study, for example in head and neck cancer. However, in certain situations free cells or tissue fragments obtained from fine-needle aspiration (FNA) biopsy can provide useful diagnostic information.

Basic audiological tests

Pure tone audiometry

This is the most commonly used investigation for hearing acuity. A pure tone audiometer delivers tones of variable frequency and intensity to the ear by either a headphone (for air conduction) or a bone oscillator placed on the mastoid process (for bone conduction). The frequencies usually tested are at octave steps, i.e. 250, 500, 1000, 2000, 4000 and 8000 Hz. Half-octave steps may also be used (3000 and 6000 Hz), especially in cases of potential noise-induced hearing loss.

> **Clinical insight**
>
> Ultrasound-guided FNA has become the cornerstone for the initial evaluation of a neck lump. Many units now have a dedicated one-stop clinic for neck lumps, where a radiologist will take the FNA specimen and a cytopathologist will examine the slides immediately to help formulate a diagnosis and management plan as part of a multidisciplinary team.

A series of short signals (tone pips) are presented at an intensity above the patient's expected threshold (the lowest-intensity sound that they can perceive) and the patient is instructed to press a button when they hear the sound. It is standard to start with 1000 Hz, with the intensity reduced in 10 dB steps until no sound is heard. The signal is then increased in 5 dB steps until half the tone pips are heard consistently, which is the threshold for that frequency. Similarly, the other frequencies are tested and plotted graphically (**Figure 2.11**). Bone conduction is similarly tested.

> **Clinical insight**
>
> When testing hearing, it is important to prevent the test sound being heard in the non-test ear. This can be achieved by the audiometer providing a continuous noise into the non-test ear, a phenomenon called masking.

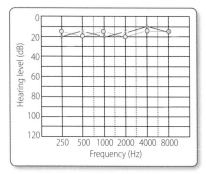

Figure 2.11 Pure tone audiogram. 'X' for left ear, 'O' for right ear air conduction. Normal hearing is generally taken as hearing threshold of 20 dB HL (hearing level) or better.

Tympanometry (impedance audiometry)

This is an objective test of middle ear function. A probe containing a sound source delivers a tone (220 Hz) into the ear, which

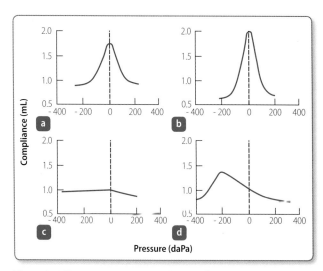

Figure 2.12 Tympanograms. (a) Normal: the peak of curve is between +50 and −100 daPa. (b) A markedly higher peak (compliance >2 mL), suggesting ossicular discontinuity. (c) A flat trace indicative of either middle ear effusion (but with normal measured ear canal volume, ECV) or tympanic membrane perforation (where there is an elevated ECV). (d) A peak with middle ear pressure of less than −100 daPa, indicative of Eustachian tube dysfunction. daPa = decaPascals.

is partly absorbed by the sound-conducting apparatus and partly reflected outwards from the surface of the tympanic membrane. The maximum absorption of sound (*compliance*) occurs when the pressures in the middle ear and the EAC pressures are equal. The probe also contains a microphone, which measures the reflected sound, and a pump attached to a manometer which enables the pressure in the meatus to be varied. *Impedance* (the resistance offered against sound passing from the tympanic membrane through the middle ear) is inversely proportional to compliance. Impedance may be increased (e.g. glue ear) or decreased (e.g. ossicular discontinuity). A tracing, reflecting the compliance, is obtained which normally shows a curve (**Figure 2.12**). The peak of this curve corresponds to the pressure in the middle ear. Normal ear pressure is between +50 and –100 decapascals.

Otology

chapter 3

The common presenting symptoms in ear disease are earache, deafness, tinnitus, vertigo and ear discharge.

3.1 Clinical scenarios

Earache (otalgia)

Background

A 21-year-old woman returned from a beach holiday with an itchy external acoustic meatus. She had used cotton buds/swabs after swimming to attempt to dry her ear. A week later she presented to her general practitioner (GP) having developed pain, crusting and erythema around the meatus and conchal bowl. She was prescribed topical antibiotic drops containing gentamicin and corticosteroids. This resulted in an initial improvement, but her symptoms returned despite continued use of the drops, and she began to develop swelling and erythema of her pinna and a purulent discharge. She returned to her GP, who sampled the discharge for microbiological culture and referred her to an otolaryngologist.

History

There is no history of immune compromise, diabetes mellitus or dermatological conditions (e.g. psoriasis).

Examination

Inspection reveals an inflamed pinna and purulent discharge at the external auditory canal (EAC) (**Figure 3.1**). Palpation reveals tenderness on manipulation of the pinna and tragus. There is mildly tender lymphadenopathy in the postauricular region. Otoscopy reveals a narrow erythematous canal filled with a purulent discharge. Otomicroscopy with microsuction reveals only a limited view of an intact tympanic membrane. Tuning fork tests indicate a conductive hearing loss.

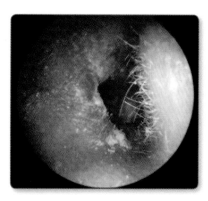

Figure 3.1 Otitis externa: erythema, oedema and crusting.

Investigation

Microbiology swab cultures of the discharge test positive for *Pseudomonas aeruginosa* (the most commonly cultured organism in otitis externa, frequently antibiotic resistant).

Differential diagnosis

- **Acute diffuse otitis externa** is usually associated with diffuse painful swelling of the EAC
- **Acute localised otitis externa** (furuncle) is associated with a localised abscess or furuncle, is excruciatingly painful and could obscure the view of the tympanic membrane, usually seen in the outer part of the EAC
- **Otomycosis** (fungal otitis externa) is common after treatment with long-term topical steroids; typical fungal infection could present with black or grey spores (*Aspergillus niger*) or creamy white discharge (*Candida albicans*)
- **Perichondritis** presents with tenderness over the pinna; once the perichondrial blood supply is compromised the cartilage may undergo avascular necrosis resulting in cauliflower ear; EAC not always involved
- **Acute suppurative otitis media** is a painful condition which may result in perforation of the tympanic membrane; the discharge contains mucus which arises from the middle ear (the EAC does not possess mucous glands)

- **Eczematous otitis externa** is usually itchy, scaly skin with eczema of the other areas and surrounding skin
- **Chronic otitis externa** is not as painful as acute infections and usually presents with a history of repeated otitis externa; skin of the external acoustic meatus is usually itchy and thickened from repeated infections
- **Osteomyelitis of the skull base** is commonly associated with diabetes and with immunocompromised status, or occurs after radiotherapy, and can involve the lower cranial nerves.

Discussion

The diagnosis here is acute diffuse otitis externa, a bacterial infection of the EAC and the most common form of otitis externa. The other types of otitis externa in the differential are acute localised, fungal and chronic forms. It is a common condition, predisposed by water ingress, warm moist conditions, immunocompromised status and diabetes, local trauma/ cerumen impaction (in this case the cotton buds) and dermatological conditions. *Pseudomonas* is the most frequently cultured organism.

Treatment involves gentle microsuction of the ear canal to remove accumulated debris and to allow better antibiotic penetration, together with topical antibiotic and steroid eardrops or ointment. Sometimes a wick is required if the canal is very swollen.

> **Clinical insight**
>
> - Repeated topical antibiotics may predispose to otomycosis (fungal otitis externa)
> - In diabetics or immunocompromised patients with long-standing 'chronic otitis externa' with pseudomonal infection recalcitrant to treatment, consider the possibility of skull base osteomyelitis. If diagnosed and treated early, one can prevent and/or limit the morbidity due to involvement of the lower cranial nerves.

Adult deafness

Background

A 34-year-old white woman presented to her GP with bilateral hearing loss, which had been progressively worsening over the previous few years. She had noticed it had worsened more rapidly during her recent pregnancy. She was finding it more difficult to hear people on the phone with her right ear and had swapped to her left ear, which seemed less affected.

On questioning it became clear that she had mild pulsatile tinnitus in her right ear in addition to her hearing loss. Strangely, she was finding that her hearing improved in noisy environments. The GP also noticed that, considering the level of hearing impairment she was displaying, she was rather softly spoken. She was referred to her local ENT department for a hearing test and assessment.

History

There is no significant history apart from a normal pregnancy and normal full-term delivery. The patient's son is now 18 months old. She has no history of prior trauma, infection or otorrhoea. She says she has an aunt with a similar presentation of deafness who now wears hearing aids, although no further information is available about her diagnosis. She is a non-smoker and non-drinker.

Examination

On presentation to the ENT outpatient clinic she is found to have a bilateral conductive hearing loss (on Rinne's test), with a right lateralising Weber's tuning fork test. Otoscopic examination reveals intact and healthy tympanic membranes; however, a faint pinkish hue is visible behind the right tympanic membrane when viewed with a microscope.

Investigation

A pure tone audiogram shows a conductive hearing loss with an air–bone gap greater in the lower frequencies and a Carhart's notch (masked bone conduction has a dip present at 2 kHz) (**Figure 3.2**). The left ear audiogram also has features of conductive hearing loss, but not as marked as on the right side. Tympanometry shows reduced compliance of the tympanic membrane (**Figure 3.3**). Further audiological testing reveals absent bilateral stapedial reflexes.

Differential diagnosis

- **Otosclerosis** is likely if there is a conductive hearing loss with an intact and healthy tympanic membrane and no other contributory history

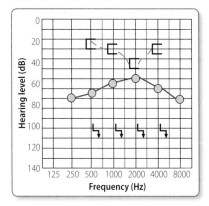

Figure 3.2 Right ear audiogram showing conductive hearing loss.

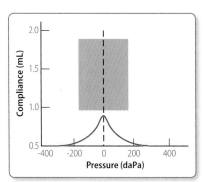

Figure 3.3 Tympanogram of right ear showing reduced compliance in otosclerosis. Shaded area indicates normal range. daPa, decaPascals.

- **Tympanosclerosis** can also present in a similar manner, especially if there is involvement of the middle ear ossicles. A chalky white plaque may be seen on the tympanic membrane
- **Ossicular discontinuity** is usually a result of previous infection, with necrosis of part of the ossicular chain (most often the long process of the incus); rarely the ossicular chain can be disrupted by traumatic injury
- **Otitis media with effusion** gives variable otoscopic findings, with a dull, retracted, grey or featureless tympanic membrane and loss of the cone of light; sometimes air bubbles

or a fluid level in the middle ear can be visualised through a thin tympanic membrane

- **Ménière's disease** in its early stages can present with a low-frequency sensorineural hearing loss; episodic rotatory vertigo, aural fullness and tinnitus are other characteristic features of this disease
- **Malleus and/or incus ossicular fixation** can be due to middle ear tympanosclerosis (above), usually with tympanic membrane involvement, or congenital fixation
- **Congenital cholesteatoma** is a rare condition in which epithelial rest cells in the temporal bone form a cholesteatoma; it presents as a white lesion in the middle ear, behind an intact tympanic membrane.

More rarely, consider:

- Glomus tympanicum tumour: a vascular swelling in the middle ear
- Paget's disease can thicken skull bones to affect hearing conduction acoustically or neurologically
- Osteogenesis imperfecta (van der Hoeve syndrome) can cause hearing impairment, usually through ossicle fracture or deformity. Presentation is commonly with a blue sclera and a history of multiple fractures
- Ankylosing rheumatoid arthritis affecting the incudostapedial joint usually presents with a history of other joints being affected.

Discussion

The diagnosis here is **otosclerosis.** The disease process has a genetic basis and sometimes the hearing loss worsens during pregnancy. In the early stages a pinkish tinge of the tympanic membrane (Schwartz's sign) may be seen, imparted by dilated blood vessels on the promontory. More often the tympanic membrane looks normal. Conductive hearing loss with a Carhart's notch on pure tone audiometry, low

Clinical insight

Most causes of conductive hearing loss are generally amenable to surgical treatment at a later stage, whereas sensorineural hearing loss and tinnitus are generally permanent or improve partially.

compliance on tympanometry and absent stapedial reflexes are features highly suggestive of fixity of the stapes footplate, which is associated with the diagnosis of otosclerosis. Management of this condition is mainly surgical (stapedectomy).

Vertigo

Background

A 55-year-old woman developed a mild upper respiratory tract infection with a runny nose and sore throat. A few days later she woke up with the sensation that the room was spinning around her. When she tried to get up it worsened, and when she tried to walk she veered off to the right, but was able to walk without falling over. Over the next few hours her symptoms worsened. She felt nauseated and vomited twice. She stayed in bed with her head still and eyes closed for the rest of the day. Her husband called the GP, who prescribed cyclizine 50 mg three times daily. After taking this her symptoms improved a little, and gradually abated over several days. Over the following months she continued to have occasional episodes of imbalance.

History

The patient has type 2 diabetes mellitus and hypercholesterolaemia. She smokes 10 cigarettes per day. She takes simvastatin and gliclazide regularly.

Examination

When the GP arrived the patient was lying still in bed, on her side with her eyes closed. Examination revealed spontaneous nystagmus with the fast phase to the left, which persisted in every direction she looked, but diminished when she fixed her gaze. When her head was rapidly rotated to the right (head thrust test), catch-up saccades to the left to realign her gaze with the midline were noted (due to loss of the vestibulo-ocular reflex). She was generally unsteady when performing Romberg's test. An Unterberger's test caused her to rotate to her right. A full neurological examination was otherwise unremarkable. The tympanic membranes were normal. Weber's test was central and Rinne's test was positive bilaterally.

Investigation

The patient is seen in the ENT clinic several weeks later. A pure tone audiogram is normal. Caloric testing reveals canal paresis on the right. She has risk factors for a stroke. An MRI scan of the brain and internal auditory meatus is normal.

Differential diagnosis

- **Acute vestibular failure** (e.g. vestibular neuritis) is associated with vertigo, nausea and vomiting without hearing loss and tinnitus
- **Cerebellar infarction** presents with common and non-specific symptoms such as dizziness, nausea and vomiting, unsteady gait and headache
- **A first episode of Ménière's disease** may lack all of the classic features of hearing loss, dizziness and tinnitus
- **Migrainous vertigo** should be considered in the presence of headaches
- **Labyrinthine infarction** occurs when the internal auditory artery is blocked, resulting in loss of auditory and vestibular function
- **Multiple sclerosis** can cause vertigo, with lesions in the brainstem, cerebellum and cerebrum.

Discussion

The diagnosis here is acute vestibular failure secondary to a viral vestibular neuritis. Treatment is supportive and conservative. Vestibular sedatives may be required in the early stages to prevent significant associated nausea and vomiting, but should be avoided long-term as they will hinder recovery. Admission and intravenous fluids may be required if fluids cannot be kept down orally. The worse effects of the vertigo usually last up to 3 weeks.

Ear discharge (otorrhoea)

Background

A 68-year-old woman developed a progressively worsening left-sided otalgia over 3 months associated with purulent, occasionally bloodstained otorrhoea. Initially her GP tried two courses of antibiotic/steroid ear drops for a presumptive diagnosis of left otitis externa. However, her pain had recently become unbearable, uncontrolled by paracetamol and diclofenac sodium. One morning she woke up with a watery, inflamed left eye and noticed that her face had dropped on the left side. Her voice had become breathy. She promptly returned to the GP, who immediately sent her for an urgent ENT opinion.

History

The patient has diabetes, diagnosed 10 years earlier, but she is poorly compliant with her diet. She is a smoker, lives alone, and has poor personal hygiene. She takes gliclazide, metformin and aspirin regularly. She is currently taking framycetin/dexamethasone ear drops, paracetamol and diclofenac sodium.

Examination

The patient is apyrexial but looks unwell. Her left ear is full of purulent debris, and after microsuction the external acoustic meatus is seen to be generally oedematous. There is some granulation tissue along the posteroinferior external acoustic meatus. The tympanic membrane is intact. Formal examination of the cranial nerves reveals a lower motor neuron left facial palsy, absent gag reflex and left tongue weakness (**Figure 3.4**). Flexible nasal endoscopy reveals a paralysed left vocal fold. There is some tenderness around the left temporomandibular joint.

Investigation

The relevant investigations are summarised in **Table 3.1**.

Clinical insight

Investigating vertigo:

- Establish exactly what happened during the first episode
- Note associated otological or neurological symptoms
- The duration of vertigo can help differentiate the underlying cause: benign paroxysmal positional vertigo (BPPV) episodes usually last a few minutes; whereas Ménière's disease episodes can last hours and those of acute vestibular failure days
- The degree of nystagmus can help in monitoring resolution in acute vestibular failure. Initially patients may have third-degree nystagmus (present looking in all directions), but as they improve the nystagmus shifts to second-degree (present looking in the direction of the nystagmus and straight ahead) then to first-degree (only present looking in the direction of the nystagmus)
- Vestibular rehabilitation exercises facilitate central brain vestibular compensation.

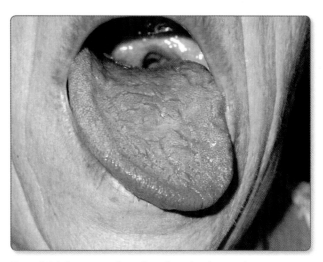

Figure 3.4 Left tongue weakness due to hypoglossal nerve palsy.

Differential diagnosis

- **Necrotising 'malignant' otitis externa** causing osteonecrosis of the temporal bone and involving multiple cranial nerves at the skull base
- **Osteoradionecrosis of the temporal bone** (after radiotherapy) with similar clinical features to necrotising otitis externa
- **Malignancy** (primary from squamous cell carcinoma of external ear canal or secondary, e.g. local spread from parotid malignancy)
- **Progressive chronic otitis media** with squamous disease (e.g. cholesteatoma)
- **Granulomatous condition of the middle ear**, e.g. Wegner's granulomatosis, sarcoidosis or histiocytosis X.

Discussion

The diagnosis here is necrotising 'malignant' otitis externa. Multidisciplinary team discussion is highly recommended in cancer cases to review radiological, histological and microbiological

Investigation	Findings
Full blood count	WBC 15 x 10^9/L (neutrophilia)
C-reactive protein	153 mg/L (normal <10)
Glucose – random glucose test	23 mmol/L
Pure tone audiogram	Moderate mixed hearing loss in left ear
Microbiology (left ear swab)	Heavy growth of *Pseudomonas aeruginosa*
Histology (biopsy of granulation tissue left external acoustic meatus)	Chronic inflammation
CT of temporal bones and chest with contrast	Bony destruction of left external acoustic meatus and mastoid extending to the skull base and temporomandibular joint. Chest normal
MRI of neck and head with gadolinium	Widespread soft tissue inflammation around the left temporal bone, stylomastoid and jugular foramen, extending to the adjacent hypoglossal canal, left infratemporal fossa and left temporomandibular joint. Brain normal

Table 3.1 Results of investigations in a woman with otalgia

investigations prior to planning definitive treatment. Treatment principles include careful microsuction of the affected ear to remove infective debris, careful diabetic control, good nutrition to assist wound healing, and topical and systemic antibiotics (e.g. ciprofloxacin). In general, surgery is not indicated although local debridement may aid recovery. Adjuvant hyperbaric oxygen treatment can be considered.

Clinical insight

- Ear pain and discharge in an elderly diabetic patient must be considered to be necrotising otitis externa until proved otherwise, and promptly investigated and treated to avoid further spread of the disease

- Antibiotics should be prescribed in line with local antibiotic policy and after discussion with the consultant microbiologist, as long-term treatment will be necessary

- A gallium-67 radioisotope scan is useful in monitoring disease activity and resolution.

3.2 Otitis externa

Otitis externa is an infective condition with associated inflammatory changes to the lining of the external acoustic meatus. It can be localised (commonly referred to as a furuncle) or diffuse, affecting the canal and the surrounding skin.

Epidemiology

Otitis externa is one of the commonest otological conditions encountered in clinical practice, with a lifetime incidence of 10% in the general population. It is associated with swimming, diving and warm and humid climates. It affects all age groups, with a peak incidence in 5–16-year-olds.

Causes

The causes of otitis externa include:
- Local irritation of the external acoustic meatus skin due to constant exposure to water
- Minor trauma to the external acoustic meatus skin secondary to cotton bud use or ear syringing for impacted wax
- Bacterial infection, the most common pathogens being *Pseudomonas aeruginosa* and *Staphylococcus aureus*
- Fungal infections such as *Candida* are common.

Hot and humid weather can exacerbate the condition.

Pathogenesis

The outer two thirds of the lining of the external acoustic meatus contain sebaceous and ceruminous glands, secretions from which help to maintain an acidic environment, which protects against infection. A paucity of cerumen – or indeed excess secretions – can create an environment that encourages bacterial multiplication. Any localised trauma that breaches the epithelial layer of the skin can lead to an invasion of pathogenic organisms, causing infection and the typical associated inflammatory reaction.

Clinical features

Symptoms are dependent upon the extent of disease and hence quite variable. Patients usually present with severe otalgia, discharge, and occlusion of the external acoustic meatus due to inflammatory oedema. The otalgia may be exacerbated by jaw opening and manipulation of the pinna. In severe cases there may be cellulitis of the surrounding soft tissues and secondary perichondritis of the pinna.

Diagnostic criteria/investigation
Otitis externa is a clinical diagnosis made after a thorough history and examination. The signs of inflammation and debris within the external acoustic meatus are usually diagnostic. Swabs of the pus and debris sent for culture and sensitivity are usually the only investigation needed. In case of recurrent/chronic otitis externa regular monitoring of inflammatory markers may be useful to assess the prognosis. A biopsy and CT scan of the temporal bones may be required in suspected cases of necrotising otitis externa.

Differential diagnosis
- **Otorrhoea** from middle ear infection can be the cause of otitis externa
- **Skin conditions** – seborrhoeic dermatitis, atopic dermatitis and psoriasis
- **Foreign body** in the external acoustic meatus, particularly in children
- **Necrotising otitis externa** – infection of the external canal skin and osteomyelitis of the underlying temporal bone in immunocompromised patients such as diabetics
- **Referred pain** originating from teeth, throat and temporo-mandibular joint
- **Ramsey Hunt syndrome** – herpes zoster infection affecting the geniculate ganglion, presenting with facial palsy and vesicles in and around the external acoustic meatus, including the tympanic membrane.

Management
- Regular aural toilet to remove the debris by microsuction is the mainstay of treatment

Clinical insight
Examination of the tympanic membrane can be obscured in otitis externa by an oedematous EAC. As there are no mucous glands in the EAC, if pus is observed in the canal it should be presumed that the tympanic membrane is perforated.

- Topical ear drops containing antibiotics and steroids (commonly used combinations are gentamicin plus hydrocortisone and framycetin plus dexamethasone)
- An ear wick expands the external acoustic meatus and also allows delivery of the ear drops in patients with an occluded meatus (**Figure 3.5**)
- Systemic antibiotics may be required when there are signs of cellulitis, perichondritis and necrotising otitis externa
- Incision and drainage might be required in furunculosis.

Repeated use of antimicrobial and steroidal ear drops may predispose to fungal otitis externa even in immunocompetent patients. It is important to give antifungal topical medication for at least 3 weeks, as fungal spores germinate later and sporicidal medication needs to continue even after the fungal hyphae have been dealt with. Microsuction and aural toilet are useful in cleaning the debris and ensure that the topical agents have access to the affected area.

Prognosis

Otitis externa is often self-limiting and the majority of cases resolve without complications. Elderly, diabetic and other immunocompromised patients require close observation, as they can develop necrotising otitis externa, which requires further investigations and aggressive treatment.

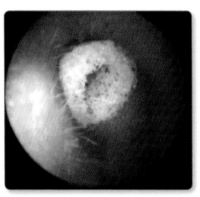

Figure 3.5 An expanded ear wick in the external acoustic meatus.

3.3 Acute otitis media

Acute otitis media is an infective inflammation of the middle ear cleft (**Figure 3.6**). It occurs in conjunction with other systemic symptoms. There are three types:

- Non-suppurative: resolves before the stage of suppuration
- Suppurative: tympanic membrane perforates with suppurative discharge
- Recurrent: three or more acute episodes of otitis media in 6 months, or more than four episodes in 12 months.

Epidemiology

Acute otitis media is one of the commonest diseases in children, with a peak incidence between 6 and 11 months. By the age of 3 years 50–85% of children have had acute otitis media. By the age of 7 years very few children still experience acute otitis media. Adults constitute approximately 16% of cases.

Causes and pathogenesis

Predisposing factors are summarised in **Table 3.2**.

Usually an antecedent viral infection causes inflammation of the middle ear mucosa and disruption of Eustachian tube

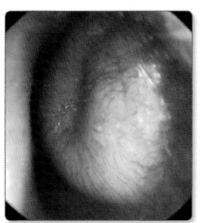

Figure 3.6 Bulging tympanic membrane due to acute otitis media.

Factor	Effect on incidence
Age	First attack before the age of 6 months is a strong risk factor for recurrent episodes
Gender	Higher incidence in males
Race	Commoner in Native Americans, Canadians, Alaskans and Australasians
Exposure to other children	Attendance at day-care facilities is major risk factor, as is exposure to other siblings at home
Cigarette smoke	Passive smoking causes inflammation of mucosa of middle ear cleft and impaired mucociliary function
Seasonal variation	More common in winter months
Genetics	Recurrent acute otitis media seems to be associated with genetically determined immunoglobulin markers
Breastfeeding	Protective effect by virtue of immunologic and antibacterial components of breast milk
Use of dummies/pacifiers	Higher incidence when used

Table 3.2 Predisposing factors for acute otitis media

function. Middle ear effusion provides a favourable medium for bacterial pathogens, which travel from the nasopharynx via the Eustachian tube. Organisms invade the mucosa of the middle ear cleft, resulting in oedema, exudate and pus. The Eustachian tube is blocked with oedematous mucosa and the pressure from the exudate tenses and bulges the tympanic membrane; in some cases the membrane perforates, which relieves the pressure and the majority of cases resolve within a week.

Common viruses are respiratory syncytial virus (RSV), parainfluenza, rhinovirus, influenza, enterovirus and adenovirus. When bacterial superinfection results, the commonest pathogens are *Streptococcus pneumonia* (35%), *Haemophilus influenza* (25%) and *Moraxella catarrhalis* (15%).

Host factors

Various factors predispose to infections in children, e.g. a shorter, more horizontal and more pliable Eustachian tube; and in children with cleft palate impaired function of tensor veli palatini predisposes to a higher incidence. Nasopharyngeal colonisation with potential middle ear pathogens does not usually cause acute otitis media owing to local mucociliary clearance and innate and adaptive immunity – lysozyme, lactoferrin, immunoglobulin (Ig) A, IgM and IgG. A breakdown of any of these host factors can lead to overwhelming infection. The role of adenoids in pathogenesis is unproven.

Clinical features

The clinical features are summarised in **Table 3.3**. Approximately 10% of patients have a discharge at presentation.

Management
Analgesics and watchful waiting

Symptomatic treatment with analgesia and antipyretics is essential. In healthy children older than 2 years with non-severe illness (mild illness, fever < 39° C) adequate analgesia may be all that is needed.

Symptoms	Signs
• Earache – from slight in mild cases to throbbing and severe; the pain is relieved if the tympanic membrane perforates • Irritability/sleep disturbance – a child may cry or scream • Otorrhoea • Deafness – conductive type • Tinnitus	• Fever – the child may be flushed and ill, high fever (up to 40° C) • Tenderness may be present around mastoid • Tympanic membrane on otoscopy – red and congested in early stages; if untreated progressively becomes tense and bulging (**Figure 3.6**) and may perforate with discharge of pus

Table 3.3 Clinical features of acute otitis media

Antibiotics

High-dose amoxicillin is the drug of choice (80–90 mg/kg/day). Amoxicillin–clavulanic acid (40 mg/kg/day amoxicillin component) is second-line treatment.

In cases of allergy to penicillin (non-IgE) cefuroxime 50 mg/kg/day is used. In selected cases, macrolides such as azithromycin or clarithromycin may be an option. Treatment duration varies from 1–2 weeks.

Surgical treatment

Surgical methods include:
- **Myringotomy** Recommended for impending complications, severe illness, failure to respond to antibiotics and to aid microbiological diagnosis
- **Tympanostomy tube** For children with recurrent acute otitis media this reduces the number of episodes
- **Adenoidectomy** May reduce the number of episodes/need for tympanostomy tube replacement after they fall out; benefits greater in children over 2 years old. Risks include haemorrhage and transient velopharyngeal insufficiency.

> ## Clinical insight
> - In a child the ear perforation usually heals quickly once acute otitis media resolves
> - Ear drops are not helpful with an intact ear drum, however they can be used for a short duration with a perforated tympanic membrane.

Prognosis

The incidence of complications is low – 1:1000 in untreated infection in children and 0.25/100 000 in adults. The incidence increases in children younger than 2 years, with recurrent acute otitis media, in patients with underlying predisposing factors and in those with severe clinical symptoms. Complications are summarised in **Table 3.4**.

Sequelae include:
- Hearing loss
- Perforation of tympanic membrane
- Chronic/adhesive otitis media
- Ossicular discontinuity/fixation.

Complication	Notes
Intratemporal	
Mastoiditis	Commonest complication Treatment with intravenous antibiotics, myringotomy or urgent cortical mastoidectomy depending upon initial response/presentation
Subperiosteal abscess	Treatment with incision and drainage with or without cortical mastoidectomy
Facial nerve palsy	Very rare Treated with myringotomy and intravenous antibiotics Approximately 95% resolve completely
Labyrinthitis	Bacterial labyrinthitis usually leads to a dead ear
Intracranial	
Meningitis	Commonest intracranial complication Relatively uncommon in adults
Lateral sinus thrombosis	This is best imaged by MRI scan
Brain abscess	Will require neurosurgical input
Otic hydrocephalus	Suspect if headache and signs of raised intracranial pressure

Table 3.4 Complications of acute otitis media

3.4 Chronic otitis media

Chronic otitis media is a persistent or recurrent inflammation or infection of the middle ear cavity. It can be classified as active or inactive, mucosal or squamous (cholesteatoma), or healed.

Epidemiology

Chronic otitis media is a common condition with a prevalence of 4%, increasing to 12% in the healed group in the UK. It affects both genders equally, with a higher prevalence in lower socioeconomic groups and manual workers.

Causes and pathogenesis

The causes of chronic otitis media are similar to those of acute otitis media, being multifactorial in origin. Negative middle ear pressure due to Eustachian tube dysfunction, upper respiratory tract infections, craniofacial abnormalities, autoimmune disease and immune deficiency all lead to middle ear disease. Although chronic suppurative otitis media may follow an initial acute infection, the pathogens are different from those found in acute suppurative otitis media. The most common organisms include *Pseudomonas aeruginosa*, *Proteus* species and *Staphylococcus aureus*. Other less common organisms include *Escherichia coli*, *Streptococcus pneumoniae*, diphtheroids, *Klebsiella* and anaerobic *Bacteroides* species.

Clinical features

The majority of patients with active mucosal or squamous chronic otitis media (cholesteatoma) will present with hearing loss (~80%), otorrhoea (~70%), and otalgia (~40%), usually with a background history of childhood ear disease. **Figure 3.7** demonstrates a posterior tympanic membrane perforation with middle ear keratin.

Approach to the patient

Chronic otitis media is definitively diagnosed on otoscopy; however, the history should focus on otological symptoms, severity

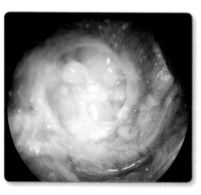

Figure 3.7 Cholesteatoma.

and previous management. Care should be taken if vertigo is present, as this may point to labyrinthine complications such as a fistula in the lateral semicircular canal (LSCC). Mandatory microscopic examination of the ear assesses for scars (end- or postaural), EAC, mastoid cavity (granulations, keratin), tympanic membrane (perforation, retraction (**Figure 3.8**), tympanosclerosis), middle ear (ossicles, effusion (**Figure 3.9**), active infection or squamous disease.

Investigation

Pure tone audiometry with air and bone conduction (with masking) complemented clinically by tuning fork tests assesses the degree of hearing impairment. Tympanometry is useful to confirm middle ear pressures. Microbiological swabs should be taken to identify aerobic and anaerobic pathogens. Vestibular assessment is performed, with a fistula test for LSCC fistula. CT of the temporal bones with 1.5 mm sections in both coronal and axial planes will aid surgical anatomy and foresee bony complications prior

> ### Clinical insight
>
> Inspect the 'attic' region of the eardrum for a pit, retraction or keratin (suggestive of cholesteatoma). This is easily missed unless you have adequate illumination, the right sized speculum and have approached the ear at the correct angle. Foul-smelling intermittent discharge with periodic flare-ups is the common presenting sign of a cholesteatoma.

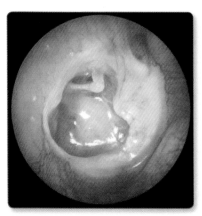

Figure 3.8 Adhesive process showing severe retraction of the tympanic membrane (right ear).

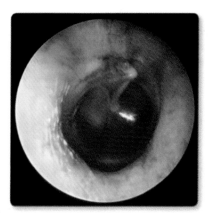

Figure 3.9 Serous otitis media (right ear).

to surgical management. MRI is useful to delineate intracranial pathology that may complicate chronic otitis media.

Management

The main principles in managing chronic otitis media are to:

- obtain a dry ear
- prevent recurrent infection
- minimise hearing loss.

Whether the disease is active or inactive, mucosal or squamous, or healed will determine the modality of treatment.

Conservative measures to dry the ear are frequent aural toilet under microscope, the application of appropriate topical antibiotic/steroid ear drops, eradicating concurrent upper respiratory infection, and preventing water entering the EAC. The commonest topical antibiotic agents are the aminoglycosides, with gentamicin, framycetin and neomycin being common constituents of aural preparations. Topical ciprofloxacin or ofloxacin have been used for *Pseudomonas* infection. Corticosteroids such as hydrocortisone and dexamethasone help reduce inflammation.

Active squamous chronic otitis media (cholesteatoma)

Here the mainstay of treatment is surgical excision of the disease, with reconstruction of the hearing mechanism at a later stage.

This can be performed by a variety of methods but essentially requires mastoidectomy (either canal wall up, canal wall down, combined approach or atticotomy) and tympanoplasty. The principal aim of treating cholesteatoma is to remove the disease and eliminate the risk of major complications.

Complications

Extracranial complications include:
- Otitis externa
- Myringitis
- Ossicular erosion (especially the long process of incus)
- Tympanosclerosis
- Middle ear adhesions
- Labyrinthine fistula
- Labyrinthitis
- Facial nerve paralysis
- Petrositis
- Acute mastoiditis.

Intracranial complications include:
- Bacterial meningitis
- Extra- or subdural abscess
- Cerebellar or temporal lobe abscess
- Sigmoid sinus thrombophlebitis.

3.5 Facial palsy

Dysfunction of the facial nerve results in facial weakness, leading to considerable functional and cosmetic impairment. It can be classified by:
- cause
- site (central versus peripheral)
- speed of onset
- extent (partial or complete).

The course and branches of the facial nerve are shown in **Figure 3.10** and **Table 3.5**.

Causes

Important causes of facial palsy are tabulated in **Table 3.6**. Paralysis can be caused by pathology anywhere along the

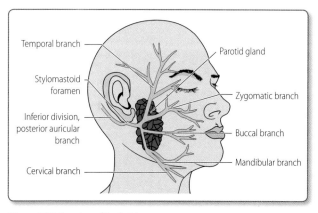

Figure 3.10 Branches of the facial nerve.

Nerve segment	Course and branches
Intracranial segment, from brainstem to internal auditory canal	Motor root and nervus intermedius (parasympathetic and sensory root) join to form common facial nerve at point of entry to an internal auditory canal
Meatal segments	Within internal auditory canal
Labyrinthine segment	Ends at geniculate ganglion; greater superficial petrosal nerve branches off at the first genu
Tympanic (horizontal) segment	Runs across the middle ear to the second genu; the most common site of dehiscence
Mastoid (vertical) segment	Runs to the stylomastoid foramen where it exits the skull. The branches to stapedius and the chorda tympani are given off here
Extratemporal segment	3 small branches (posterior auricular, nerve to the stylohyoid, nerve to posterior digastric) followed by pes anserinus where nerve divides into its final 5 branches (temporal, zygomatic, buccal, mandibular, cervical)

Table 3.5 Course and branches of the facial nerve

Aetiology	Important causes
Upper motor neuron (supranuclear and nuclear)	Intracranial tumours, vascular lesions (e.g. stroke), multiple sclerosis
Lower motor neuron	
Infectious/idiopathic	Idiopathic facial paralysis, herpes zoster oticus, necrotising otitis externa, otitis media/ mastoiditis, Lyme disease, meningitis
Trauma	Temporal bone fractures, penetrating facial injuries
Tumours	Cholesteatoma, cerebellopontine angle lesions (including vestibular schwannoma and meningiomas), parotid tumours

Table 3.6 Aetiology of facial nerve palsy

course of the nerve. Supranuclear or upper motor neuron fibres (cortical nerves which control the nucleus) will often spare the forehead, as they receive fibres from both facial nerve nuclei.

Clinical features

Facial nerve paralysis is devastating for the patient as it affects the ability to smile, frown and express emotions. Facial movement is asymmetrical and the patient is unable to close his eyes tightly, puff out his cheeks, clear food from inside the cheek, show his teeth or whistle. He also may drool from one side, have an impaired sense of taste (if the lesion is above the origin of the chorda tympani nerve) and have reduced tear production if the lesion is above the geniculate ganglion, where the greater superficial petrosal nerve arises. Reduced lacrimation can lead to loss of the blink reflex and corneal damage.

Investigation

Investigations are summarised in **Table 3.7**.

Type of test	Description
Electrodiagnostic	
Electromyography	The facial nerve is stimulated adjacent to the stylomastoid foramen. The evoked electromyographic activity from the facial muscles is measured: >90% early degeneration suggests poorer prognosis for recovery of facial function
Topographic	
Schirmer's test (tests tear production) Stapedial reflex test Saliva production test	These have largely been replaced by electrodiagnostic tests

Table 3.7 Investigations in facial palsy

Management
Idiopathic facial paralysis (Bell's palsy)

Idiopathic facial nerve paralysis (palsy) or Bell's palsy is diagnosed after all possible causes of facial palsy have been ruled out. It constitutes the vast majority (60%) of facial nerve palsies seen and is believed to be a viral cranial neuritis most often caused by herpes simplex type I (HSV-I). The clinical feature is rapid onset (<48 hours) and it may be associated with a viral prodrome, hyperacusis, decreased lacrimation and taste disturbance. One third present with weakness (paresis) and two thirds with loss of movement (paralysis).

Treatment should start promptly, preferably within 24 hours. Oral prednisolone (1 mg/kg/day, up to 60 mg daily) is the treatment of choice, tapered over a 2 week period. Eye care with lubricants and

Clinical insight

The Scottish Bell's Palsy Study (2007) concluded that early treatment with prednisolone significantly improved the chances of complete recovery at 3 and 9 months. There was no evidence of a benefit from acyclovir given alone or of any additional benefit from acyclovir given in combination with prednisolone.

Facial palsy in acute or chronic otitis media requires urgent referral to an ENT surgeon for possible surgery.

an eye pad at night is an important aspect of management, and 80% patients make a full recovery. In the remaining 20% thorough investigations, including CT or MRI and electrodiagnostic tests (**Table 3.7**), help with the prognosis and future management.

Herpes zoster oticus (Ramsay Hunt syndrome)

This is a primary infection or reactivation of herpes zoster virus in the geniculate ganglion. Clinical features include the features of Bell's palsy, with vesicles on the tympanic membrane, external acoustic meatus and palate (**Figure 3.11**). The patient is usually elderly, and pain may precede the facial palsy. This may affect other cranial nerves – rarely IX, X, and very occasionally V, VI or XII. Management is similar to that for Bell's palsy. In addition, antivirals (e.g. aciclovir) may improve the prognosis and reduce postherpetic neuralgia.

The prognosis is not as good as in idiopathic facial paralysis as only 60% make a full recovery.

Iatrogenic injury

The tympanic and mastoid segments are at risk in otologic surgery; the extratemporal segment is at risk in salivary gland surgery, with facelifts and with neck dissections. A transected nerve can be reanastomosed or cable grafted at the

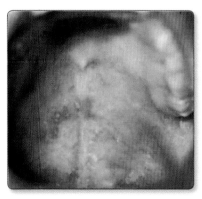

Figure 3.11 Palatal vesicles as a manifestation of herpes zoster (Ramsay Hunt syndrome type II).

time of or soon after surgery. A nerve weakness (neuropraxia) or delayed paralysis usually recovers fully. Oral steroids may offer some benefit.

3.6 Otosclerosis

Otosclerosis is a localised disease of the otic capsule. It is a disorder of bone remodelling and clinically manifests as conductive hearing loss. It has a predilection for the oval window (fissula ante fenestrum), though other areas are less commonly involved.

Epidemiology

Otosclerosis is more common in the white population. Prevalence is similar in both sexes, though females manifest with a higher degree of hearing loss. Pregnancy is thought to accelerate the progression of disease. In approximately 75% of cases the disease is bilateral.

Causes

The exact cause is unknown, but current theories include:
- Genetic predisposition: autosomal dominant with incomplete penetrance
- Measles: there is some evidence for an association
- Autoimmunity to type II collagen: although the evidence is weak.

Sporadic cases, where there is no family history, have also been described.

Pathogenesis

In otosclerosis there is a region (focus) of increased bone turnover with osteoclastic and osteoblastic activity. The initial focus is otospongiotic, with resorption of bone, enlargement of perivascular spaces and deposition of immature bone. Eventually the disease burns out with deposition of dense lamellar bone, known as an otosclerotic focus. The commonest area of involvement is anterior to the oval window. This leads to progressive fixation of the stapes circumferentially in the region of the annular ligament, and sometimes involves the entire footplate. The result is conductive hearing loss. Sensorineural hearing loss may also occur as a consequence of involvement of the spiral ligament.

Clinical features
- Gradually progressive asymmetric conductive hearing loss, often with a family history of otosclerosis.
- Quiet speech, as patients are able to hear their own voice
- Paracusis – the ability to hear better in noisy surroundings is seen in the early stages
- Tinnitus and rarely dizziness or vertigo.

Investigation
- Pure tone audiometry – conductive hearing loss; characteristically a 'Carhart's notch' is seen – a dip in bone conduction at 2 kHz (see **Figure 3.2**)
- Tympanometry – normal in the early stages, although with progression the compliance decreases
- Stapedial reflexes – these will be absent
- A high-resolution CT scan can be helpful – a hypodense area is seen anterior to the oval window, with thickening of the stapes footplate.

Diagnosis and differential diagnosis

Clinical otosclerosis is a presumptive diagnosis. Otoscopy reveals an intact tympanic membrane. Rarely, a 'flamingo flush' or 'Schwartz sign' is seen: a red blush of the tympanic membrane due to an active, vascular focus of otospongiosis over the promontory. A history of progressive conductive hearing loss along with these

Clinical insight

In an adult who presents with a conductive hearing loss with a normal eardrum, otosclerosis is a likely diagnosis. In about three-quarters of patients the disease is bilateral.

The diagnosis is presumptive based on clinical assessment and complemented by audiological tests. The diagnosis is confirmed in those patients who are treated surgically by performing a surgical exploratory tympanotomy and checking for stapedial fixity.

findings is highly suggestive of the diagnosis, though the gold standard is demonstrating stapes fixation intraoperatively.

Differential diagnosis

The differential diagnosis includes the following more common disorders:

- Ossicular discontinuity
- Tympanosclerosis
- Malleus and/or incus ossicular fixation
- Otitis media with effusion
- Adhesive otitis media

Rare differentials are:

- Glomus tumour
- Middle ear tumour
- Paget's disease
- Congenital footplate fixation
- Osteogenesis imperfecta (van der Hoeve syndrome)
- Ankylosing rheumatoid arthritis.

Management

Reassurance and review If hearing loss is unilateral or mild and the patient does not have significant disability a repeat audiometric assessment may be arranged.

Hearing aid

Amplification with hearing aids gives good results and a trial prior to surgery is a reasonable option. A bone-anchored hearing aid (BAHA) has also been proposed as an option.

Medical

Sodium fluoride is used to slow the progression of disease. It is contraindicated in patients with chronic nephritis, or chronic rheumatoid arthritis, in pregnant and lactating women, and in children and in those with allergy to fluoride. However, evidence for its use is not robust.

Surgery

Surgery (stapedectomy) is the best method of treatment for otosclerosis and produces dramatic improvements in hearing if it is successful, though there is a high price to pay in the event of failure (around 1%).

Stapedectomy is most commonly performed, though many variations can be used. A tympanomeatal flap is elevated to gain access to the middle ear and stapes. Stapes fixation is confirmed. A prosthesis is placed through an opening in the vestibule through the stapes footplate (**Figure 3.12**), attaching it to the incus, thereby improving sound conduction through the ossicles. Lasers can also be used for stapes surgery to create the fenestra in the footplate – potassium titanyl phosphate (KTP), argon and CO_2 laser have also been used. Postoperatively patients are advised to avoid activities such as lifting heavy objects, flying, diving, parachuting and contact sports.

Risks of surgery There is a risk of severe sensorineural hearing loss postoperatively – reported to be 1–4% for primary surgery. Tinnitus is unlikely to improve and may worsen after surgery; taste sensation can be affected if the chorda tympani nerve is stretched or damaged, and vertigo is usually a transient feature.

Prognosis

Stapedectomy is a specialised procedure and generally performed by dedicated and skilled otologists. Success rates for improving hearing are around 95%.

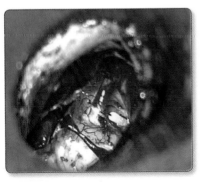

Figure 3.12 Stapes prosthesis in position.

3.7 Presbyacusis

Presbyacusis (also known as presbycusis) is a progressive sensorineural hearing loss associated with age (Greek *presbys* = *elder* and *akuein* = *to hear*). The progressive degeneration with age results in reduction in acuity of hearing, especially in the higher frequencies, and difficulty in discrimination of speech in old age.

Epidemiology

It affects up to 50% of people over the age of 55 and the prevalence is equally distributed between males and females.

Causes and pathogenesis

The cause is largely uncertain but there are several theories:

- Atrophy of epithelial tissue in the basal turn of the cochlea, resulting in a reduction in the number of hair cells
- Atrophy of neural tissue in the spiral ganglion cells causing loss of neurons
- Atrophy of the stria vascularis caused by vascular disorders
- Loss of elasticity of the basilar membrane due to degeneration of the spiral ligament
- Chronic noxious stimuli such as noise.

Factors that may aggravate or accentuate presbyacusis include atherosclerosis, diabetes, noise trauma, smoking, dietary habits (increased intake of saturated fats), hypertension and ototoxic drugs (e.g. aspirin), and the condition may have a genetic basis.

Clinical features

Progressive sensorineural hearing loss, usually bilateral and symmetrical, affects the hearing frequencies over 1 kHz, creating a typically downward sloping audiogram. The patient finds it hard to hear high-pitched sounds, such as birdsong, alarm bells, TV and radio, and has difficulty in discriminating speech, especially in the presence of background noise. Tinnitus sometimes accompanies the hearing loss.

Investigation

Pure tone audiometry displays increasing sensorineural bilateral hearing loss in frequencies of 1000 Hz upwards (**Figure 3.13**). MRI might be required if there is any asymmetry between the right and left side hearing thresholds. Blood tests to exclude other causes of premature deafness include FBC, urea and electrolytes, lipids, TFTs, ESR, ANCA, ACE, tissue autoantibodies and viral serology.

Diagnosis

The diagnosis is based on history, depending on the patient's age, the appearance of the audiogram and exclusion of other causes.

Management

Sound amplification via hearing aids is the best method of treatment. The patient needs to make their family and friends aware of the handicap so that they can assist by speaking slowly but not too loudly, facing the patient. Lip-reading skills are useful. Occasionally rehabilitation in the form of auditory training and hearing therapy is required to allow the patient to cope better with the hearing loss and/or tinnitus. Accessory aids using induction coils fitted to telephones and televisions are also helpful.

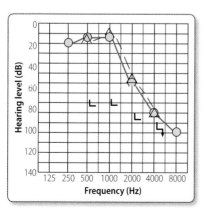

Figure 3.13 Audiogram showing right high-frequency sensorineural hearing loss.

Prognosis

With modern digital hearing aids most presbyacusis patients cope well. The hearing loss might progress, requiring appropriate adjustment of hearing aids.

3.8 Ménière's disease

Ménière's disease is an inner ear disorder characterised by episodes of vertigo, fluctuating sensorineural hearing loss, tinnitus and aural fullness.

Epidemiology

The incidence is approximately 50–150 cases per 100 000 people per year. It is more common in women and tends to present in the fourth or fifth decade of life; 30–40% develop bilateral disease.

Causes and pathogenesis

Excess endolymph production results in dilatation of the membranous labyrinth, known as endolymphatic hydrops. Ménière's attacks are thought to occur when the endolymphatic pressure becomes high enough to cause microtears in the membranous labyrinth, leading to mixing of endolymph with perilymph. Sometimes the endolymphatic hydrops can be attributed to a specific disease, such as mumps, syphilis, Cogan's syndrome or trauma; the clinical symptoms are then known as Ménière's *syndrome*. When no cause can be found it is called Ménière's *disease*.

Clinical features

Spontaneous attacks of vertigo, fluctuating unilateral hearing loss, tinnitus and aural fullness occur. They last hours and are associated with nausea and vomiting. Initially hearing and balance return to normal after an attack, but as the disease progresses hearing loss and dysequilibrium may persist between episodes. The disease may occasionally manifest as drop attacks with no loss of consciousness and immediate complete recovery (crisis of Tumarkin).

Investigations and diagnosis

The diagnosis is primarily clinical, based on a history of two or more episodes of vertigo with associated hearing loss, tinnitus and aural fullness. During an attack horizontal nystagmus is evident.

There is no diagnostic test. A pure tone audiogram may be normal in the early stages of the disease. A permanent sensori-neural loss then develops, initially affecting the low frequencies (**Figure 3.14**) and later affecting all frequencies equally. Blood tests to exclude other causes of hearing loss and vertigo should be performed:

- FBC for leukaemia and anaemia
- Urea and electrolytes for urinalysis (otorenal syndrome)
- Thyroid screen (TSH, T3, T4)
- CRP
- Glucose to rule out diabetes
- Lipid profile – hyperlipidaemia is known to be associated with hearing loss and vertigo
- ESR and autoantibody screen, including antineutrophil cy-toplasmic antibody (ANCA) and antinuclear antibody (ANA) for autoimmune disorders
- Venereal Disease Research Laboratory test (VDRL) for neu-rosyphillis

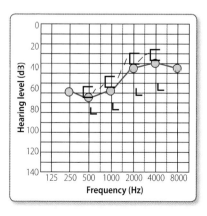

Figure 3.14 Audiogram showing right low-frequency sensorineural hearing loss.

- Viral titres for viral causes of Ménière's syndrome (e.g. measles or mumps).

MRI scanning enables the exclusion of an acoustic neuroma or other retrocochlear pathology. Caloric testing may show a reduced response from the affected side.

Management
Prevention of attacks
- Counselling and reduction of stress
- Dietary modifications include strict salt restriction (<2 g/day) to reduce endolymph accumulation, and avoidance of caffeine and alcohol to prevent rapid fluid shift
- Diuretics may prevent endolymph accumulation, e.g. bendroflumethiazide 2.5 mg daily
- Betahistine may improve vestibulocochlear blood flow
- Steroids may be administered via the oral or the intratympanic route during an active phase of disease
- Intratympanic gentamicin administration controls vertigo by chemical ablation of the vestibular apparatus, but may also cause permanent hearing loss; it must therefore be used with care if there is serviceable hearing because of the risk of bilateral Ménière's disease developing.

Relief of symptoms during attacks
Vestibular sedatives, e.g. cinnarizine and prochlorperazine, are useful during an attack, however they should not be continued after the attack subsides as they suppress normal vestibular activity and prevent vestibular compensation and recovery.

Medical management of long-term effects
The following all have a role in the long-term management:
- Hearing aids
- Vestibular rehabilitation exercises
- Tinnitus retraining therapy.

Surgical management
This is indicated when symptoms remain uncontrolled despite optimal medical therapy. Options include the insertion of

grommets, but the mechanism of their action is unknown. The Meniett device can be used after grommet insertion. It delivers low-pressure pulses to the ear which are thought to displace perilymph, resulting in increased flow of and subsequent reduction in endolymphatic fluid. Endolymphatic sac decompression aims to reduce endolymphatic hydrops, but results are variable and it is performed less frequently than in the past. Vestibular nerve section stops attacks of vertigo but does not improve hearing or tinnitus symptoms. Surgical labyrinthectomy involves destruction of the entire labyrinth and controls vertigo at the expense of any remaining hearing.

Prognosis

The disease tends to follow a relapsing and remitting course. Some patients have few attacks and no permanent sequelae, whereas others are afflicted by rapidly progressive disease with frequent severe attacks and debilitating vestibular insufficiency, tinnitus and hearing loss.

3.9 Benign paroxysmal positional vertigo

Benign paroxysmal positional vertigo (BPPV) is defined as an abnormal sensation of motion elicited by certain critical provocative positions. It is the most common cause of vertigo; other causes are listed in **Table 3.8**.

Causes and pathogenesis

Predisposing factors for BPPV are:

- Inactivity
- Acute alcoholism
- Head injury
- Major surgery
- CNS disease.

It is caused by an abnormal movement of calcified crystals (otoliths) in the semicircular canals. There are two theories as to how vestibular sensation is disordered by the crystal collections to cause BPPV:

Cause	Characteristics
Benign paroxysmal positional vertigo	Most common cause; head movements cause a feeling of motion
Ménière's disease (section 3.8)	Accompanied by tinnitus and hearing loss
Vertebrobasilar insufficiency	Lack of blood to base of the brain causes momentary attacks, usually not associated with ear symptoms
Ototoxic drugs, e.g. aminoglycosides	Constant vertigo with ear symptoms
Acute labyrinthitis	Severe vertigo, total loss of hearing – may be suppurative or idiopathic
Vestibular neuronitis	Solitary acute attack where cochlea is spared, aetiology may be viral or vascular
Trauma	Acute vertigo may occur after ear surgery or head injury
Multiple sclerosis	Abrupt onset
Migraine	Usually followed by headache
Acoustic neuroma	With unilateral tinnitus and hearing loss

Table 3.8 Common causes of vertigo

- *Canalithiasis* – free moving concretions in the posterior semi-circular canals cause disordered endolymph movement
- *Cupulolithiasis* - abnormal dense particles attached to the cupula cause a disordered response of the (heavy) cupula to endolymph movement.

Classic BPPV involves the posterior semicircular canal (SCC). Abnormal particle movement in the semicircular canal causes mismatch of sensory information, which results in the sensation of vertigo.

Clinical features

Classic BPPV is characterised by the sudden onset of transient (seconds to minutes) true spinning vertigo triggered by changes in head position (bending down, looking up, turning to one side). In extreme cases slight head movement can cause vertigo and vomiting. Generally the attacks will stop or improve after a few weeks or months, but in some cases they can persist for longer.

The nystagmus associated with BPPV has several important characteristics that differentiate it from other types of nystagmus:

- Triggered by changes in head position
- 5- to 10-second delay in onset and lasts for 5–120 seconds
- Visual fixation does not suppress nystagmus
- A rotatory/torsional component or (in the case of lateral canal involvement) the nystagmus beats in either a geotropic (towards the ground) or an ageotropic (away from the ground) fashion
- Fatiguability on repeated stimulation.

Investigation and diagnosis

The condition is diagnosed from the patient's history (feeling of vertigo with sudden changes in positions) and by performing **Hallpike's manoeuvre (Figure 3.15)**, which is diagnostic for the condition:

- This test is performed by rapidly moving the patient from a sitting to a supine position with the head turned 45° to the right
- After approximately 20–30 seconds the patient is returned to the sitting position
- If no nystagmus is observed the procedure is then repeated on the left side.

In a positive test, during the supine phase there is fast rotatory (torsional) nystagmus of the eye towards the affected ear, with nystagmus in the opposite direction after returning to the seated position.

The finding of classic rotatory nystagmus with latency and limited duration is considered pathognomonic for BPPV. A negative test cannot rule out BPPV. A complete otoneurological examination is necessary to rule out other vertiginous disorders.

Management

Vertigo usually subsides either spontaneously or with the assistance of vestibular exercises and balance therapy.

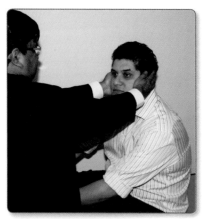

Figure 3.15 Hallpike manoeuvre. The patient is rapidly moved from sitting to a supine position with the head turned 45° to the right and returned to the sitting position after 20–30 seconds. Both sides are tested. A positive test shows nystagmus of the eye towards the affected ear when supine, with nystagmus in the opposite direction after returning to the seated position.

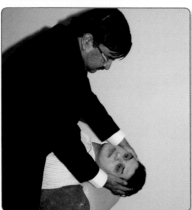

Conservative or watchful waiting

Spontaneous remission can occur within 6 weeks, although some cases never remit.

Canalith repositioning

This is the first-choice treatment. It aims to move particles from areas in the inner ear which cause symptoms (the semicircular canals) and reposition them where they do not (vestibule of the vestibular labyrinth). Various methods exist; the two most established being the Epley and Semont manoeuvres. Each takes about 15 minutes to complete and can often give immediate and long-lasting relief from BPPV.

Epley's manoeuvre

- Starts with the patient sitting, head turned 45° towards the ipsilateral side
- Turn head 90° to the other side
- Roll the body onto the side with head in the same direction, so the nose is pointing down
- Finally, return the patient to sitting with the head tilted down slightly.

The interval between positions is 30–60 seconds, based on the duration of the vertigo and nystagmus. This procedure can be repeated.

The Semont manoeuvre This is performed by the patient turning rapidly from lying on one side to the other. It is generally considered both more difficult and more uncomfortable for the patient.

Brandt–Daroff home exercises These involve a precise sequence of moving from a sitting position to specific lying positions and need to be repeated several times a day for 2–3 weeks.

Rotational chair and home devices These rotating-chair devices enable a patient to perform particle repositioning at home, usually similar to the Epley sequence.

Medications Medical treatment with antivertigo medications may be considered in acute severe exacerbations of BPPV, but in most cases are not indicated.

Prognosis

BPPV is a self-limiting condition. Epley's manoeuvre has a success rate of more than 95%, the recurrence rate varying between 10% and 25%.

3.10 Sudden sensorineural hearing loss

This is a sensorineural hearing loss of 30 dB or more in three or more adjacent frequencies over a period of up to three days. It is nearly always unilateral.

Epidemiology

The incidence is thought to be between 2–20 cases per 100 000 people per year. The true incidence is not known, as in many cases the hearing returns to normal before the patient sees a doctor. It is most common in the fifth and sixth decades of life, but can occur at any age.

Causes and pathogenesis

The majority of cases are idiopathic. There are many theories about the aetiology which centre mainly around vascular occlusion, viral infection, autoimmunity and intracochlear membrane ruptures. In a few cases there is an identifiable cause; common ones are listed in **Table 3.9** and must be sought in all patients.

> **Clinical insight**
>
> - Acute-onset sensory neural hearing loss is an otologic emergency and treatment, albeit empirical, should be instituted without delay
> - Bilateral profound sensorineural loss is devastating but the majority of patients recover to some extent.

Causes	Examples
Infection	Viral – herpes simplex, varicella zoster, mumps, measles, rubella Bacterial – meningitis, syphilis
Tumour	Acoustic neuroma, leukaemia, myeloma
Trauma	Temporal bone trauma, barotrauma, noise trauma, iatrogenic
Ototoxic drugs	Aminoglycosides, loop diuretics, salicylates
Ménière's disease	Associated with an acute attack
Central cause	Multiple sclerosis, stroke
Systemic disease	Hypothyroidism, diabetes, hyperlipidaemia, sarcoidosis, autoimmune disorders including Cogan's syndrome, Wegener's granulomatosis, polyarteritis nodosa, systemic lupus erythematosus

Table 3.9 Common causes of sensorineural hearing loss

Clinical features

The patient often reports waking up with hearing loss. In other cases hearing rapidly deteriorates over several hours. There may be associated tinnitus or vertigo.

Weber's test localises to the side opposite to the affected ear and Rinne's test is positive in the affected ear. The external auditory meatus and tympanic membranes are normal. Ear wax does not cause hearing impairment unless it is impacted against the tympanic membrane and causes conductive rather than sensorineural hearing loss.

Investigation

This aims to confirm the diagnosis, quantify the magnitude of the hearing loss and identify a cause, with a view to providing appropriate treatment.

- Drug history, particularly salicylates, diuretics, aminoglycosides, antimalarials, cisplatin, and beta-blockers
- Pure tone audiometry to confirm a sensorineural hearing loss and assess the severity
- Tympanometry confirms normal middle ear pressure and excludes an effusion
- Haematology: FBC for infection and polycythaemia; ESR for autoimmune disease; clotting for coagulopathy
- Biochemistry: glucose for diabetes mellitus; lipid profile for hyperlipidaemia; thyroid function tests for hypothyroidism; ANCA for Wegener's granulomatosis; ACE for sarcoidosis; autoantibody screen
- Serology: syphilis serology; viral titres
- MRI enables the exclusion of acoustic neuroma or central pathology.

> ## Clinical insight
>
> Unilateral or asymmetric sensorineural hearing loss must be investigated to rule out an acoustic neuroma. Although usually the onset is gradual and insidious, in a small minority the presentation can be acute and sudden. MRI of the internal auditory meatus with gadolinium enhancement is the gold standard. Early diagnosis reduces mortality and morbidity.

Management

Any reversible cause identified should be treated appropriately. The management of idiopathic hearing loss is an area of great controversy and there is little evidence for any of the treatments available. Treatment is aimed at improving cochlear microcirculation. Steroids are most commonly used, e.g. oral prednisolone 30–60 mg daily for 7 days; intratympanic steroids are gaining popularity to mitigate side effects. Antivirals are also in widespread use, e.g. aciclovir 800 mg five times a day for 10 days. Other options include carbogen gas, betahistine and hyperbaric oxygen. Vasodilators and plasma expanders are no longer commonly used.

Prognosis

Complete remission occurs spontaneously in approximately 50% of patients. Full recovery is thought to be less likely when:
- The hearing loss is associated with vertigo
- There is a severe to profound loss
- The audiogram is downward sloping.

Hearing aids should be provided for those with persistent moderate to severe hearing loss.

3.11 Acoustic neuroma (vestibular schwannoma)

A vestibular schwannoma (acoustic neuroma) is a benign tumour of the Schwann cells of the vestibular portion of the eighth cranial nerve (**Figure 3.16**). The widely used term 'acoustic neuroma' is in fact a misnomer.

Epidemiology

Vestibular schwannomas (VS) account for approximately 8% of intracranial tumours and for 80% of cerebellopontine angle lesions. The incidence is 10 per million per year. The usual age of presentation is from 40 to 60 years.

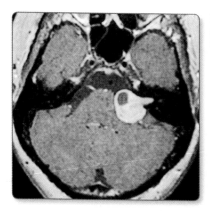

Figure 3.16 MRI showing gadolinium enhancement of an acoustic neuroma.

Causes and pathogenesis

Five per cent of vestibular schwannomas are inherited (as neurofibromatosis type (NF2) or familial vestibular schwannoma), the remainder are sporadic.

Schwannomas arise from a mutation in the gene coding for a tumour suppressor protein called Merlin. It is inherited in an autosomal dominant fashion; patients with NF2 inherit one abnormal Merlin encoding gene and appear to develop schwannomas when a mutation occurs in the second allele.

Clinical features

The typical presentation is with asymmetric sensorineural hearing loss, often high frequency and associated with tinnitus. This can be progressive or sudden in onset. There can be vestibular disturbance in the form of impaired balance or vertigo.

A more advanced case may also present with signs of facial nerve compression resulting in facial paresis. Hitselberger's sign is hypoaesthesia of the conchal bowl and external acoustic meatus.

Other higher cranial nerves (V, IX, X, XI) may be involved. With larger tumours patients may present with intracranial symptoms of ataxia, headache and raised intracranial pressure.

Investigation

Investigations and clinical findings are summarised in
Table 3.10.

Management

The treatment modality and surgical approach are selected
based on tumour size and growth, comorbidities and level of
hearing. In small tumours observation with serial MRI scans is
recommended, as 50% have very little if any growth.

Stereotactic radiation therapy is a highly localised form of
radiotherapy that inhibits growth and reduces collateral injury.
This form of treatment is typically for small tumours (<2–3 cm
diameter) and poor surgical candidates.

Surgical approaches include:

- Translabyrinthine – sacrifices hearing but otherwise lower
  morbidity, hence used where hearing is already lost
- Retrosigmoid – preserves hearing, higher morbidity
- Middle cranial fossa – preserves hearing, limited to small
  tumours.

Prognosis

The main risks of surgery are hearing loss, facial nerve palsy,
intracranial infection and/or haemorrhage. Intracranial procedures carry a 1% mortality rate.

Investigations	Findings
Pure tone audiogram (PTA)	Unilateral or asymmetrical sensorineural loss
Speech discrimination	Disproportionate poor speech discrimination
Auditory brainstem-evoked response (ABR)	Increased latency between N1 and N5 waves
Vestibular tests	Reduced or absent caloric responses
Imaging	Gadolinium enhancement on MRI (see **Figure 3.16**)

Table 3.10 Investigations and findings in patients suspected of having acoustic
neuroma

3.12 Trauma to the ear

Trauma may affect the external, middle or inner ear or a combination of these, and present with symptoms depending on the severity and the region affected. It may be as a result of direct, indirect or blunt trauma (**Table 3.11**).

Severe injuries can result in fractures of the temporal bone. Temporal bone fractures are classified into:

- Longitudinal (parallel to the temporal bone axis)
- Transverse (right-angles at 90° to temporal bone axis)
- Oblique (combination of the two).

Pathogenesis

External ear trauma

Usually in the form of a laceration with or without cartilage involvement or a pinna haematoma; this can result in avascular necrosis of the cartilage leading to a *cauliflower ear*, as the blood supply to the perichondrium is compromised when it is stripped from the underlying cartilage. Cauliflower ear creates a cosmetic deformity and is best avoided by early intervention.

Middle ear trauma

This can result in perforation of the tympanic membrane, haemotympanum (blood collection in the middle ear) or ossicular chain discontinuity.

Region	Causes
External ear	Direct impact: foreign bodies, cotton buds, iatrogenic, syringing, sports injury (rugby)
Middle ear	Barotrauma (acute pressure change caused by forceful Valsalva, diving, flying, explosions), iatrogenic, insertion of sharp foreign bodies (e.g. hairpins)
Inner ear	Direct impact: missiles or sharp instruments, severe trauma leading to fractures of temporal bone Indirect impact: blast injuries/explosions, loud noise

Table 3.11 Common causes of ear trauma

Inner ear trauma

Inner ear trauma involving fracture of the temporal bone can affect the vestibule, cochlea, semicircular canals, facial nerve and round and oval windows.

Clinical features

The clinical features of trauma to the ear are shown in **Table 3.12**.

Longitudinal temporal bone fractures create a combination of haemotympanum, Battle's sign (postaural bruising), conductive hearing loss, distortion of the meatal anatomy and rarely vestibular signs. Transverse fractures usually cause sensorineural hearing loss, facial nerve injury, vertigo, nystagmus and possible CSF otorrhoea.

Investigation

Ear trauma is usually diagnosed with a full and thorough history correlated with appropriate clinical assessment. In the case of middle and suspected inner ear trauma, thorough examination of the ear under microscopy is required. Hearing assessment

Region	Clinical presentation
External ear trauma	Bleeding Pain
Middle ear trauma	Conductive deafness Perforation of the tympanic membrane Haemotympanum (bleeding into the middle ear) Transient tinnitus or vertigo
Inner ear trauma	Conductive or sensorineural deafness Vertigo Tinnitus Nystagmus Facial nerve paralysis Cerebrospinal fluid otorrhoea (rare)

Table 3.12 Clinical features of traumatic injury to the ear

carried out clinically and confirmed with a pure tone audiogram distinguishes between conductive and sensorineural hearing loss. Imaging studies (CT scan) are required to investigate the possibility of a temporal bone fracture (**Figure 3.17**).

Management
External ear trauma
If sharp, requires thorough cleaning or debridement and suturing of the skin alone (not the cartilage), with precise approximation of the helix edge if this has been severed. A pinna haematoma or abscess requires aspiration if small, or formal incision and drainage, pressure application (head bandage or suturing a dental roll through the ear) and the administration of appropriate antibiotics (usually quinolones when cartilage injury is suspected).

Middle ear trauma
Early management is usually conservative. This requires systemic antibiotics, and rarely myringotomy and drainage of any blood clots (haemotympanum) is needed. Traumatic perforation of the tympanic membrane requires review by an ENT specialist after a few weeks to assess the degree of damage and plan for any required surgery.

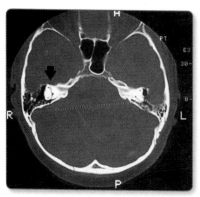

Figure 3.17 CT scan showing transverse temporal bone fracture.

Inner ear trauma

Inner ear trauma is usually treated conservatively after ensuring there is no other intracranial damage. A combination of anti-biotics and steroids is administered, and possibly a vestibular sedative in case of vertigo. Facial nerve trauma is an area of debate in terms of early or late surgical intervention, and the involvement of a specialist otologist is advisable.

Rhinology

4.1 Clinical scenarios

Nose bleed (epistaxis)

Background

A 79-year-old man presented to his GP with a 3-week history of nose bleeds. The initial episode lasted for 45 minutes and settled with conservative measures. Since then, he had noticed intermittent nasal bleeds whenever he blew his nose. His most recent episode started in the early hours of the morning and continued for over 3 hours, affecting predominantly the left nostril. He was unsure about blood running down inside his throat. His GP suggested that he visit the local emergency department for ENT assessment and further management.

History

The patient has hypertension, controlled by appropriate medication. He has ischaemic heart disease and had a coronary artery bypass graft (CABG) 12 years ago. He has been on statins and low-dose aspirin (75 mg) for the last 5 years. He had two courses of antibiotics following an upper respiratory tract infection last winter. His cardiologist started him on anticoagulants about 3 months ago.

Examination

Anterior rhinoscopy reveals blood clots in the left nostril. As there is evidence of fresh bleeding the clots are gently removed. Nasal endoscopy assessment is carried out after instilling local anaesthetic into the nose. This reveals a leash of blood vessels (a collection of vessels centring on an apex) in Little's area of the septum (**Figure 4.1**). The nasal mucosa is hyperaemic and bleeds to touch. No clots are seen in the posterior nasal cavity, and there is no evidence of any posterior bleed.

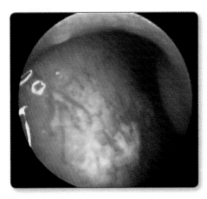

Figure 4.1 Epistaxis. Endoscopic view of the Little's area of the septum.

Investigation

Full blood count reveals a marginally low haemoglobin and normal platelet count. Coagulation studies confirm a raised INR and prolonged prothrombin time. On arrival the patient is anxious, and his blood pressure is high on initial assessment, settling with a low-dose anxiolytic (given as there was no posterior nasal bleed). The bleeding is controlled by endoscopic-guided nasal cautery with silver nitrate applied to Little's area. Self-dissolving nasal packing is then inserted in the nostril.

Differential diagnosis

Systemic causes include:

- **Hypertension**
- **Drugs**, e.g. warfarin, heparin, aspirin
- **Haematological disorders**, e.g. haemophilia, thrombocytopenia
- **Elevated venous system pressure**, e.g. mitral stenosis
- **Liver disease** and excessive alcohol use.

Local causes include:

- **Nasal trauma**, e.g. nose picking, blunt or sharp injury
- **Inflammation**, e.g. rhinitis, sinusitis, Wegener's granulomatosis

- **Drugs**, e.g. steroid nasal spray
- **Tumours**, e.g. sinonasal malignancy
- **Environmental**, e.g. temperature, humidity, altitude.

Discussion

In this case the cause of bleeding is likely to be multifactorial, with anxiety, hypertension and anticoagulant therapy playing a role in the aetiology of anterior epistaxis. The initial bleeding was controlled by local treatment with endoscopic-guided nasal cautery. In a proportion of elderly patients the nasal bleeds can recur, and a multidisciplinary team approach involving community nurses, GP, care-of-the-elderly physician, haematologist, cardiologist and the ENT surgeon plays a role in the management of the condition.

> **Clinical insight**
>
> - Anterior epistaxis is amenable to cautery, whereas posterior epistaxis is more troublesome to control and needs posterior packing
> - Vestibulitis is common in children and application of combined chlorhexidine hydrochloride and neomycin sulphate cream is sometimes all that is needed
> - In the elderly, discuss with the physician whether anticoagulants can be stopped temporarily.

Nasal obstruction

Background

A 45-year-old man went to his GP for left-sided nasal obstruction with anosmia and loss of taste, which was triggered by a bout of upper respiratory tract infection 6 weeks before. There was a background history of long-standing bilateral nasal obstruction and rhinorrhoea. The GP noticed a swelling in the left nasal cavity and referred the patient to ENT for further management.

History

The patient is asthmatic and suffers from hay fever, with a history of hypersensitivity to aspirin.

He uses inhalers for asthma and over-the-counter medication for hay fever. He is a carpenter by profession, with a 20-year history of smoking.

Examination

Anterior rhinoscopy reveals caudal deviation of the septum to the left side, with a pale, fleshy swelling in the nasal cavity which was insensitive to gentle probing (**Figure 4.2**). The mucosal lining of the nasal cavity is hyperaemic, with mucoid discharge along the floor. Nasendoscopy reveals multiple pale fleshy swellings bilaterally in the middle meatus.

Investigation

Skin-prick allergy tests reveal positive results to house dust mites, grass pollens and moulds.

A CT scan of the nose and paranasal sinuses confirms bilateral polyposis with involvement of the underlying ethmoid and maxillary sinuses. There is no evidence of underlying bony erosion. An UPSIT test (University of Pennsylvania Smell Identification Test) reveals moderate hyposmia.

Differential diagnosis

- **Rhinitis with nasal polyposis:** allergic polyps are pale, fleshy outpouchings of the sinus mucosa which are usually insensate. They most commonly originate from the middle meatus and can be 'circumnavigated' with a nasal probe
- **Rhinitis with inferior turbinate hypertrophy:** polypoidal nasal turbinates are commonly mistaken for nasal polyps;

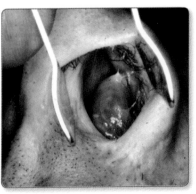

Figure 4.2 Anterior rhinoscopy revealing a left nasal polyp.

they are pale pink swellings attached to the lateral nasal wall. Sensate and highly vascular, they shrink on application of a topical nasal decongestant
- **Rhinitis with deviated nasal septum:** a common cause of nasal blockage. The septum, best visualised on anterior rhinoscopy, can block either side or both when 'S'-shaped
- **Tumours of the nasal cavity** are usually unilateral and can present with bleeding and signs related to involvement of surrounding structures (e.g. orbit involvement causing diplopia, gum involvement with loosening of teeth)
- **Cystic fibrosis:** a genetic disorder affecting multiple systems caused by an abnormality of ciliary function. The history is suggestive of chest or other organs being affected
- **Young's syndrome:** encompasses a combination of bronchiectasis, rhinosinusitis and reduced fertility.

Discussion
The diagnosis is allergic rhinitis with nasal polyposis. A thorough history with particular note of any allergy or atopy, any seasonal variation, duration and progress of symptoms, specialist assessment with nasal endoscopy, and appropriate investigations including allergy tests and imaging studies helps to establish the cause of nasal obstruction. Often the causes overlap, and a structural pathology such as septal deviation could be present, with allergic causes such as nasal polyps compounded further by infective pathology if the sinus drainage is blocked. Remember, the same respiratory epithelium lines the nasal cavity and extends to the chest; ask specifically for any coexisting chest symptoms.

Clinical insight
- **Unilateral nasal polyp** can be a large inflammatory polyp arising from the maxillary sinus and blocking the posterior choana, called antro-choanal polyp, or rarely due to sinister neoplastic origin. The primary modality is surgical excision, either for cure or for a histological diagnosis
- **Bilateral nasal polyps** are usually multiple, arising from the ethmoidal sinus, and are of allergic aetiology. Management includes medical therapy initially with intranasal steroids, allergen avoidance, antihistamines and oral steroids; surgery is reserved for extensive polyposis.

Loss of sense of smell (hyposmia)
Background
An otherwise fit and well 42-year-old woman was referred to the ENT department by her GP because she lacked the ability to smell. A full history revealed a sudden onset of symptoms following a road traffic accident 6 months earlier; this failed to improve with time. She had normal function prior to the accident. At the time of the accident she was admitted to hospital and spent a week being managed conservatively for a stable skull fracture.

Her loss of smell seemed to be complete, but she could still sense something when she used her perfume; she could also still taste things but with no sense of flavour. At the time of her accident this was a minor symptom, but she now wants it investigated. She denied any other associated symptoms such as nasal blockage, rhinorrhoea or facial pain. A trial of topical nasal steroids (fluticasone nasal spray 200 µg once daily) did not help.

History
The patient has a history of rhinitis of pregnancy. She is a non-smoker with moderate alcohol intake. There is no family history of disorder of smell.

Examination
At the outpatient clinic she is given a Sino-Nasal Outcome Test-22 Questionnaire and scores a total of 7/110. Anterior rhinoscopy reveals no abnormality and rigid nasal endoscopy shows a mild left-sided deviation of the nasal septum but no mucopus or polyps. A brief neurological examination including cranial nerve assessment is normal except for the lack of smell. The remainder of the examination, including the neck and oral cavity, is unremarkable. Unfortunately, the clinic does not have the equipment for specific olfactory testing, but in a simple test the patient can still sense an alcohol wipe when it is waved in front of her nose with her eyes closed.

Investigation

A full blood count, lipid profile, renal, liver and thyroid functions organised by the GP are all essentially normal. Skin-prick testing shows a mild response to house dust with a strong positive control. An MRI scan of the brain and skull base shows irregularity around the olfactory bulb and cribriform plate area, but no evidence of neoplasm; changes are consistent with previous trauma.

Differential diagnosis

- **Sensorineural hyposmia** (damage to the olfactory neurosensory epithelium or nerve) following viral upper respiratory tract infection, meningitis and trauma
- **Conductive hyposmia** (obstruction preventing the odoriferous molecules reaching the olfactory epithelium) of rhinosinusitis, with or without nasal polyposis
- **Central hyposmia** following a cerebrovascular accident or tumours affecting the frontal lobes
- **Iatrogenic** following intracranial procedures and endoscopic approaches to the skull base
- **Drug-induced hyposmia or dysosmia** e.g. due to zinc gluconate, carvedilol, varenicline and various chemotherapy agents.

Discussion

The diagnosis here is sensorineural hyposmia secondary to head trauma. Recovery can occur in up to 40% of patients between 6–24 months after the injury. However, this is less likely with an associated skull base fracture. Olfactory loss due to trauma is more commonly seen after frontal blows, although an occipital blow is more likely to give rise to anosmia. Recovery occurs in <10% after trauma, with most occurring within 6 months, although there have been reports of some return of smell up to 7 years after the event.

Damage to olfactory receptor neurons can also result from long-term use of vasoconstrictor nasal sprays. It would be prudent to ask specifically about this, as sometimes rhinitis of

Guiding principle

Anosmia: no sense of smell

Hyposmia: reduced sense of smell

Hyperosmia: increased sensitivity to odours

Parosmia: distorted sense of smell

Cacosmia: perception of an unpleasant odour when a normal odour presented

Phantosmia: perception of an odour in the absence of an olfactory stimulus.

Clinical insight

It is important to counsel patients with anosmia about using smoke alarms in the home.

pregnancy can be problematic and the sufferer becomes dependent on such a spray to relieve distressing symptoms.

Facial pain

Background

A 42-year-old woman is referred to the ENT outpatient clinic by her GP. She had complained of facial pain affecting the malar regions bilaterally, expanding over the maxillary sinus areas, the bridge of the nose, the orbits and radiating to the frontal regions. It started 2 years ago, occurring on a daily basis and lasting several hours, or sometimes most of the day. Her GP prescribed oral diclofenac and co-codamol, which initially offered partial relief but had recently ceased to be successful. The patient enjoyed a good night's sleep each night but described the pain as troublesome and debilitating and said she was unable to concentrate. She described a feeling of 'heaviness' over her eyes and nose, felt that her 'sinuses are blocked' and that her face 'swells up'.

Six months after first presenting, her GP diagnosed sinusitis and prescribed co-amoxiclav and fluticasone nasal spray for 14 days, but this was not successful. She was then referred to a different ENT department, where she had bilateral antral washouts. This also did not relieve the symptoms.

She denied nasal obstruction, rhinorrhoea, epistaxis or hyposmia.

History

The patient has a history of migraines, for which she takes sumatriptan. Her mother also suffers with headaches. She is a single mother, unemployed, and looks after 2 children aged

5 and 7. She admits to being under considerable stress as she is currently trying to obtain financial support from her ex-husband.

Examination

The patient's facial appearance is unremarkable. Mild tenderness is elicited by pressure over both malar regions. Anterior rhinoscopy and fibreoptic nasendoscopy are both normal. The oral cavity, dentition, alveoli and oropharynx are also normal. The findings of a clinical neurological examination are normal.

Investigations

A CT scan of the sinuses is negative for occult disease.

Differential diagnosis

Differential diagnoses to consider in this situation are:
- Midfacial segment pain
- Acute/chronic rhinosinusitis
- Migraine
- Tension headache
- Cluster headache
- Pain of dental origin/phantom toothache
- Temporomandibular dysfunction syndrome
- Post-traumatic pain
- Paroxysmal hemicrania
- Myofascial pain
- Neuralgias (trigeminal, glossopharyngeal, postherpetic)
- Tumours
- Atypical facial pain
- Temporal arteritis.

Discussion

The diagnosis here is midfacial segment pain. This is a symmetrical sensation of pressure or tightness across the midface. Symptoms of tension-type headache can coexist. The treatment in-

Clinical insight

- Facial pain in the majority of cases is not due to sinus disease
- A thorough examination including nasal endoscopy is essential to rule out a space-occupying lesion
- Pain originating from the sinuses is usually intermittent and associated with other nasal symptoms.

volves low-dose amitriptyline (10–20 mg at night), which may take up to 6 weeks to work. Alternative medication includes gabapentin.

4.2 Rhinitis

Rhinitis describes an inflammation of the nasal mucous membranes. It may be allergic or non-allergic in origin. Non-allergic rhinitis can be further classified into infective (rhinosinusitus) and non-infective (hyper-reactive nasal airway). Infective rhinitis is considered in the following section. Allergic rhinitis may be seasonal or perennial, depending on the responsible allergen. Common allergens include grass pollen, tree pollen, house dust mites, *Aspergillus*, cat allergens, dog allergens and feathers.

Epidemiology
Up to 25% of the population suffer from non-allergic rhinitis and 15–25% from allergic rhinitis. The prevalence is thought to be equal between men and women, but can vary greatly both within and between countries.

Causes and pathogenesis
Allergic rhinitis is a type 1 hypersensitivity reaction mediated by IgE. When an allergen enters the nose and binds to IgE bound to mast cell surfaces, this causes both an immediate degranulation of mast cells and a subsequent late-phase prolonged inflammatory reaction. Mast cell degranulation releases stored mediators including histamine, leukotrienes and kinins causing vasodilation and leads to (late phase) recruitment of other inflammatory cells to the nasal mucosa, including eosinophils, neutrophils, lymphocytes and macrophages.

Non-allergic rhinitis has seven basic subclassifications, shown in **Table 4.1**.

Clinical features
Allergic and non-allergic rhinitis can cause nasal block, rhinorrhoea (runny nose), postnasal drip and occasional sinus or

Vasomotor	Caused by an imbalance between the parasympathetic and sympathetic nervous regulation of the nose
Infectious	Usually viral or bacterial
Occupational	Due to inhaled irritants (e.g. solvents, latex, wood dusts)
Hormonal	Pregnancy and hypothyroidism
Drug-induced	Caused directly by drugs, e.g. ACE inhibitors, beta-blockers and cocaine, or indirectly by chronic use of a nasal decongestant (rhinitis medicamentosa)
Gustatory	Predominantly after eating hot or spicy foods
NARES (non-allergic rhinitis with eosinophilia syndrome)	Probably due to abnormal prostaglandin metabolism

Table 4.1 Subclassification of non-allergic rhinitis

Eustachian tube symptoms. Allergic rhinitis can also cause sneezing, nasal itching and ocular symptoms, with red eyes and epiphora. Allergic rhinitis is often associated with asthma or eczema and a family history of atopy.

Examination reveals nasal mucosal oedema, often with exudation and enlarged turbinates.

The classification of allergic rhinitis has been changed from the traditional terms 'seasonal' and 'perennial' to 'intermittent' and 'persistent' (**Table 4.2**).

Investigation
Skin-prick testing relies on the classic 'wheal-and-flare' response to an allergen placed intradermally in the skin.
- If mast cells are sensitised to a specific allergen a reaction will rapidly be seen
- This acute-phase reaction reaches its maximum after about 10–15 minutes
- Positive (histamine) and negative controls (saline) are also used

Classification	Characteristics
Intermittent	< 4 days/week *OR* Duration < 4 weeks
Persistent	≥ 4 days/week *AND* Duration > 4 weeks
Mild	Normal sleep plus (in untreated patients): No impairment of daily activities, sport, leisure Normal work and school No troublesome symptoms
Moderate to severe	One or more of the following: Abnormal sleep Impairment of daily activities, sport, leisure Troublesome symptoms

*From the Allergic Rhinitis and its Impact on Asthma guidelines.

Table 4.2 Classification of allergic rhinitis as intermittent or persistent, and mild or moderate to severe*

- Oral antihistamines must be stopped more than 48 hours prior to allergy skin-prick testing.

Alternatively, antigen-specific IgE may be measured directly from a blood test. This is less sensitive than skin-prick testing, but can be done even in patients taking antihistamines or during pregnancy.

The SNOT (Sino-Nasal Outcome Test) is a validated disease-specific quality of life questionnaire for the assessment of rhinosinusitis and can be a useful measure of disease progression.

Where another cause is considered a blood test may be required, in particular autoantibody screens such as serum angiotensin converting enzyme levels (sarcoidosis) and ANCA (Wegener's granulomatosis).

Cross-sectional imaging may be required when suspecting sinus disease with a view to surgery, or if there are unilateral symptoms raising a suspicion of neoplasia.

Management

Management of allergic rhinitis falls into three main categories:

- allergen avoidance and environmental control
- pharmacotherapy
- immunotherapy.

Rarely surgery may be indicated to correct a significant anatomical abnormality (deviated nasal septum) or restore adequate sinus ventilation and drainage with significant associated sinus disease or nasal polyps unresponsive to medical treatment. Management of non-allergic rhinitis uses similar pharmacotherapy, but without specific allergen avoidance and immunotherapy.

First-line pharmacotherapy This includes saline nasal douching, intranasal steroids and topical/oral antihistamines. Patients must be warned that rhinitis is a persistent condition and in most cases medication is required long-term. Occasionally, depending on the history and severity of the condition, systemic corticosteroids, oral montelukast and nasal ipratropium bromide are also used.

Immunotherapy This is generally reserved for those who do not respond to more conservative treatment. It is more effective in those who are allergic to only one common allergen to which they can be desensitised. Sublingual and intramuscular routes are the most common means of administration. The risk of anaphylaxis must always be considered and appropriate supervision provided.

Prognosis

Rhinitis is not life-threatening but does have a significant impact on quality of life. Most treatment options need to be continued long term.

4.3 Chronic rhinosinusitis

Chronic rhinosinusitis (including nasal polyposis) is defined as inflammation of the nose and paranasal sinuses characterised by two or more symptoms present more than 12 weeks, and should be either nasal blockage or discharge.

Epidemiology

Chronic rhinosinusitis affects up to 15% of the population. Almost 33 000 new cases are diagnosed with nasal polyposis yearly in England and Wales.

Causes

Several factors contribute to the condition, mainly allergy to common inhalant allergens such as grass pollen (hay fever), tree pollen, dust mites, pet dander and *Aspergillus*. Chronic rhinosinusitis with nasal polyposis is particularly common among patients with asthma, aspirin sensitivity, allergic fungal sinusitis and cystic fibrosis. Other factors include immune modulation, biofilms, structural anomalies and genetics.

Pathogenesis

The most accepted index event is the narrowing or obstruction of the sinus ostia by mucosal inflammation. This disrupts mucociliary clearance and sinus ventilation, leading to changes in microflora within the sinuses (**Figure 4.3**).

Clinical features

Two or more symptoms should be present for 12 weeks or more, one of which should be nasal blockage or nasal discharge (anterior or posterior nasal drip). The other symptoms include facial pain and hyposmia. Minor symptoms include sneezing, nasal itching and itchy, watery eyes.

Examination with anterior rhinoscopy shows inflamed hypertrophied mucosa. Reduced nasal air entry can be simply demonstrated by the misting test, which involves placing a metal tongue depressor under the nose and observing the misting pattern during respiration. Nasendoscopy is important to examine the nasal cavity and lateral nasal wall for erythema, oedema, mucopus and polyps, as well as the postnasal space. See **Table 4.3** for grading of nasal polyps.

Investigation

Allergy skin-prick testing should be performed for common inhalant allergens.

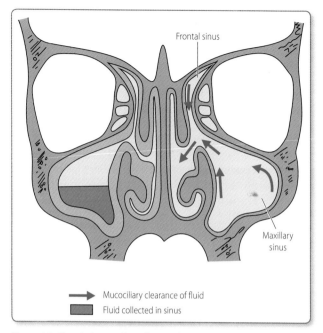

Frontal sinus

Maxillary
sinus

→ Mucociliary clearance of fluid

▇ Fluid collected in sinus

Figure 4.3 Chronic sinusitis. Normal mucociliary clearance is shown on the right side of the figure; the left side shows nasal mucosal oedema with obstruction of the ostiomeatal complex.

Grade	Description
I	Confined to the middle meatus
II	Below the level of the middle meatus but above the lower edge of the inferior turbinate
III	Causing total obstruction (below the lower edge of the inferior turbinate)

Table 4.3 Grading of nasal polyps

If a chronic inflammatory disorder is suspected, for example with significant nasal crusting, blood testing should be done for ACE (sarcoidosis) and ANCA (Wegener's granulomatosis).

> ### Clinical insight
>
> Nasal polyps in a child indicate cystic fibrosis until proved otherwise.

Bacterial and fungal cultures are of minimal clinical value in routine assessment but may have a role in investigating symptoms that persist despite medical treatment and where an unusual cause may be implicated.

CT scanning of the sinuses is reserved for patients in whom medical treatment fails, to look for anatomical abnormalities and degree of sinus involvement, and as a tool to plan surgery.

> ### Clinical insight
>
> Plain sinus radiographs have no role in the routine investigation of chronic rhinosinusitis, because abnormalities are present in up to 40% of the normal population.

The Sino-Nasal Outcome Test-22 Questionnaire (SNOT-22) is a useful measure of the impact of chronic rhinosinusitis on the individual's quality of life. It can also be used as an outcome measure of treatment.

Diagnosis and differential diagnosis

The diagnosis is made by history and clinical examination.

Differential diagnoses include acute rhinosinusitis and neoplastic conditions of the paranasal sinuses. Unilateral sinonasal disease, bony erosion or calcifications within the sinuses should raise suspicion of neoplastic disease.

Management

First-line treatment is medical, surgery being reserved for treatment failures. Treatment is summarised in **Table 4.4**.

Prognosis

Medical treatment is usually effective in controlling the symptoms in most patients. Surgery is fairly safe, but is associated with a high rate of recurrence if not followed by appropriate medical treatment and preventive measures.

4.4 Nasal polyps

Nasal polyps are pale grey pedunculated masses often prolapsing from the sinuses into the nasal cavity. They most commonly

Medical	Surgical
• Corticosteroids. Usually topical (fluticasone, mometasone, betamethasone). For severe cases, systemic steroids may be considered for short period • Saline nasal douching • Macrolide antibiotic (e.g. azithromycin or clarithromycin) for 12 weeks • Antihistamine for allergic rhinitis • Allergen avoidance and good asthma control	• Functional endoscopic sinus surgery to restore adequate ventilation and drainage of sinuses and remove polyps • Balloon sinuplasty: a relatively new procedure that can help cases with localised limited disease

Table 4.4 Treatment of chronic rhinosinusitis

arise from ethmoid air cells and less frequently from the maxillary sinuses, turbinates or septum.

Pathogenesis
Chronic inflammation of the nasal and sinus mucosa leads to oedema and reactive hyperplasia; this can progress and lead to polyp formation. There are many theories as to the exact pathogenesis, and it is incompletely understood why some people develop the disorder. In many cases the polyps are related to allergy and are sometimes attributed to chronic sinus infection, which may be bacterial or fungal. They are nearly always bilateral; if unilateral, neoplasia must be suspected. Inflammatory polyps themselves are not premalignant.

In children polyps can be related to cystic fibrosis. Asthma, aspirin sensitivity and nasal polyposis often occur together (Samter's triad).

Clinical features
Progressive nasal obstruction, rhinorrhoea, postnasal drip and anosmia are the most common symptoms.

Otological symptoms from Eustachian tube obstruction, recurrent sinusitis and occasionally headaches or facial discomfort may occur. Nasal blockage may lead to snoring and obstructive sleep apnoea. Nasal polyps may exacerbate coexisting asthma.

Rarely, distortion of the facial skeleton occurs secondary to chronic pressure from long-standing and extensive polyposis, but actual erosion of bone, either clinically or radiologically, should raise suspicion of malignancy. Inflammatory polyps are not usually bloody.

Antrochoanal polyps are less common and arise from the maxillary antrum on one side. They extend through the sinus ostium and extend posteriorly to block the posterior choana.

Investigation

Anterior rhinoscopy and nasal endoscopy should be performed. Smooth, translucent pale blue/grey pedunculated masses which can be single or multiple are seen. They are insensitive, but are usually mobile around their stalks.

Investigation of bilateral inflammatory polyps is not always necessary. If polypectomy with functional endoscopic sinus surgery is being considered, or if any sinister features such as bleeding, unilateral polyp, orbital signs and symptoms are present, then a CT scan of the sinuses including 3- to 4- mm coronal cuts should be obtained. This is used both to assess the extent and nature of the disease and as an anatomical 'road map' for endoscopic surgery.

Allergy testing by serological radioallergosorbent test (RAST) or allergy skin prick testing should be considered if suggested by the history. It's important to exclude CF in children, so a chloride sweat test or genetic testing for CF is usually indicated.

Differential diagnosis

Large polypoidal inferior turbinates may mimic nasal polyps but are vascular, sensate, and attached to the lateral nasal wall (**Figure 4.4**). Other nasal masses that may mimic the symptoms/ appearance of inflammatory nasal polyps include primary malignant tumours (usually squamous cell carcinoma – SCC), inverted papilloma, neurogenic lesions, e.g. olfactory neuro-blastoma, and juvenile nasopharyngeal angiofibroma.

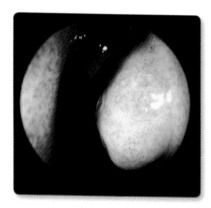

Figure 4.4 Hypertrophied nasal turbinate.

Sinonasal neoplasia may be suspected in patients having unilateral polyps with serosanguineous discharge, and nasal obstruction with or without sinus, dental or orbital symptoms. Suspected neoplasia should be investigated with both CT and MRI scanning of the sinuses for bony and soft tissue detail (see **Figure 4.8**). However, most multiple bilateral nasal polyps are benign, inflammatory or allergic in nature.

Management
Medical

Topical nasal steroid drops/sprays and/or oral corticosteroids are effective treatment for nasal polyps. Corticosteroids can be used to shrink polyps before surgery, to reduce the rate of regrowth after surgery, or as a primary treatment modality.

> ## Clinical insight
>
> Polypoidal inferior turbinates (**Figure 4.4**) can be differentiated from nasal polyps (see **Figure 4.2**) by the application of topical nasal decongestant spray, which shrinks the vascular turbinates but rarely affects nasal polyps.

Short courses of oral steroids are commonly used without significant side effects in carefully selected individuals. The effects are, however, nearly always short-lasting. A history of diabetes, TB, glaucoma, gastric ulceration/gastritis and osteoporosis are among the contraindications to this regimen.

Nasal steroid drops/sprays can shrink smaller polyps and are useful for slowing recurrence.

Some patients also show benefit from oral leukotriene receptor antagonists or macrolide antibiotics.

Surgical

This consists of polypectomy, usually together with resection of ethmoid air cells, and is nearly always performed endoscopically. A microdebrider can make this much simpler. Nasal polyps removed during surgery are sent for histology. A CT scan should be taken prior to surgery.

Prognosis

Despite surgical excision nasal polyps tend to recur, although this can be reduced by the use of long-term medical therapy (topical corticosteroid).

4.5 Epistaxis

Epistaxis is an acute haemorrhage from the nasal cavity or nasopharynx. This may be classified as anterior or posterior, depending on the location of bleeding from the nasal cavity.

Epidemiology

The lifelong incidence in the general population is around 60%, with <10% seeking medical attention. Incidence is bimodal, peaking at ages 2–10 and 50–80 years. The sexes are equally affected.

Causes

In most cases a cause is not identified; episodes tend to be self-limiting and harmless. Causes may be classified as local or general (**Table 4.5**), and include the autosomal dominant disease hereditary haemorrhagic telangiectasia (Osler-Weber-Rendu disease; **Figure 4.5**).

Pathogenesis

Bleeding typically occurs from Little's area (anterior nasal septum) in around 90% of cases, as blood vessels here are superficial and easily traumatised. This area has Kiesselbach's

Local causes	General causes
• Nasal trauma, e.g. nose picking, blunt or sharp injury • Foreign body • Nasal surgery or instrumentation • Inflammation, e.g. rhinitis, sinusitis, Wegener's granulomatosis • Drugs, e.g. steroid nasal spray • Recreational drugs, e.g. cocaine • Tumours, e.g. sinonasal malignancy, angiofibroma • Vascular, e.g. hereditary haemorrhagic telangiectasia (HHT) (**Figure 4.5**), arteriovenous malformation, endometriosis	• Hypertension • Drugs, e.g. warfarin, heparin, aspirin • Haematological disorder, e.g. haemophilia, thrombocytopenia • Elevated venous system pressure, e.g. mitral stenosis • Environmental e.g. temperature, humidity, altitude • Liver disease • Excessive alcohol

Table 4.5 Causes of epistaxis

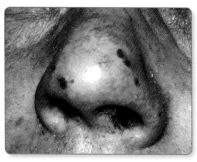

Figure 4.5 Hereditary haemorrhagic telangiectasia.

plexus of vessels, with a confluence of branches from the internal and external carotid artery systems. Posterior epistaxis usually originates from branches of the sphenopalatine artery.

Clinical features

Most anterior epistaxis presents as unilateral bleeding from the nares. In posterior epistaxis blood will also pass down into the pharynx and may compromise the airway. Blood may be spat out from the mouth and vomited up if swallowed.

If haemorrhage is severe and prolonged the patient is at risk of developing symptoms and signs of hypovolaemic shock. Recurrent epistaxis may lead to iron deficiency anaemia.

Investigation

Laboratory investigations are not normally required but are recommended for recurrent epistaxis, for major haemorrhage, or depending on the clinical picture, e.g. easy bruising suggesting a coagulopathy. Blood tests are indicated for the following situations:

- Recurrent epistaxis or patients with systemic conditions (e.g. neoplasia or platelet disorder): FBC, coagulation studies, hepatic and renal function
- Persistent heavy bleeding: FBC, haematocrit count, type and cross-match (for possible transfusion), coagulation studies
- Patients on warfarin: FBC, coagulation studies.

Diagnosis

Diagnosis is on clinical grounds, but special investigations and an appropriate specialist opinion may be required if an unusual cause is suspected.

Management

Airway, breathing and circulation (ABC)

First principles of management in the emergency setting are attention to the airway, breathing and circulation, with resuscitation as appropriate.

Conservative

The patient should be sitting up and leaning forward. Pinch the soft part of the nose and place an ice pack over the nasal bridge for 15–20 minutes. In cases of high blood pressure an antihypertensive such as amlodipine may be considered. In children and adults with self-limiting epistaxis a 2-week course of topical antiseptic (e.g. chlorhexidine and neomycin sulphate cream) and avoidance of digital trauma will often prevent recurrence. Iron deficiency anaemia should be corrected.

Once bleeding stops

Clearance of clots (reduces local fibrinolysis) by blowing the nose or by gentle suctioning with a flexible suction catheter; application of a topical vasoconstrictor with local anaesthetic (lidocaine with phenylephrine spray); examination of the nose and silver nitrate nasal cautery to any visible bleeding point on Little's area. After cautery the patient may be discharged on topical antiseptic cream.

Clinical insight

Silver nitrate nasal cautery can potentially cause perforation of the nasal septum. To reduce this risk, the septum should not be cauterised at adjacent areas on both sides.

Packing

Anterior nasal packing is indicated if bleeding does not arrest with the above measures:

- A nasal tampon (ideally lubricated with a water-based gel) should be placed into each nasal cavity
- These should be placed for 24–48 hours and the patient admitted.
- Consider broad-spectrum antibiotics (e.g. co-amoxiclav) if packs remain for more than 24 hours
- If anterior epistaxis persists, packing with layered ribbon gauze impregnated with BIPP (bismuth, iodoform, paraffin paste) should be performed.

If anterior packs fail posterior packs are indicated:

- A female (short) Foley catheter can be passed nasally until the tip of the tube is seen in the oropharynx; the balloon is inflated in the nasopharynx and gently pulled anteriorly to occlude the posterior choana. The tube is carefully secured at the nasal tip to avoid posterior migration
- Bilateral balloon packs may be required, with anterior nasal packing to occlude the nasal cavities and provide tamponade in an attempt to control the bleeding
- When a Foley catheter is secured for posterior nasal packing it is essential that a soft gauze pack is placed between

Types of ligation	Other techniques
• Endoscopic sphenopalatine artery • Maxillary artery via Caldwell–Luc • External carotid artery • Anterior and posterior ethmoidal artery	• Nasal packing under general anaesthesia • Electrocautery under general anaesthesia • Endovascular maxillary artery embolisation • Laser treatment or Young's procedure (nasal closure) for HHT

Table 4.6 Surgical management of epistaxis

the securing clip and the alar region of the nose to prevent pressure necrosis and loss of cartilage, with nasal deformity. Rarely surgery will be required (**Table 4.6**).

Clinical insight

Beware of using benzodiazepines in the elderly: they can cause sedation and risk to the airway, especially in the presence of posterior epistaxis into the pharynx.

Prognosis
Silver nitrate cautery is highly effective for an anterior bleed. Nasal packing can control the majority of more severe bleeds without long-term sequelae. Mortality is rare and associated with hypovolaemia secondary to severe bleeding, or in patients with comorbidities. Morbidity is often due to the complications of packing, including nasal obstruction, anosmia, aspiration of clots, posterior migration of the pack causing airway obstruction, perforation of the nasal septum or pressure necrosis of cartilage, and infection.

4.6 Nasal trauma

Nasal fracture is the most common facial fracture (between 40–50%) and the third most common fracture of the bony skeleton. Trauma to the nose may result in soft tissue injury, fracture or dislocation of the septum, septal haematoma, fracture of the facial skeleton and CSF leak.

Causes
Nasal fractures are commonly seen following assaults, accidents and sports injuries. In children they are common after falls.

Pathogenesis

The direction of force to the nose during injury determines the pattern of the nasal fracture. Force applied from a frontal direction may cause an infracture of the lower margin of the nasal bones (which are thinner than the heavier, upper portion). A heavier force would result in severe flattening or splaying of the nasal bones and fracture of the septum.

Lateral forces may cause a depression of the ipsilateral nasal bone, or may also be forceful enough to outfracture the contralateral nasal bone. When the nose is twisted or buckled, the fractured bony and/or cartilaginous fragments are often interlocked. This is important to identify because achieving an adequate result with a closed technique may be impossible in such a situation. The septum is often fractured and may be dislocated off the maxillary crest. Proper reduction of the septum is critical to obtaining optimum results. The fracture pattern of the septum varies according to the location of the fracture.

Clinical features

Clinical findings in patients with a history of trauma to the nose or face may result in epistaxis, swelling, deformity (**Figure 4.6**), nasal airway obstruction, and occasional infraorbital ecchymosis.

Diagnosis

A thorough examination and good history taking are vital in the diagnosis of nasal fractures. Plain radiographs are unnecessary for simple nasal fractures. A complete history should be taken of:

- The force, direction and mechanism of injury
- The presence of epistaxis or CSF rhinorrhoea
- Nasal obstruction or any abnormalities with smell or vision
- Any obvious deformity as noted by the patient
- Previous nasal obstruction and fractures, to prevent confusing previous deformities with the acute injury.

A thorough nasal examination should be performed. In a patient with no apparent abnormality at the initial visit, reassessment of the nose after 5–7 days when the oedema has subsided may reveal findings necessitating repair. The

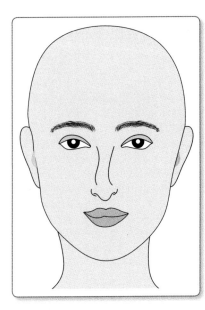

Figure 4.6 Deviation of the upper two-thirds of the nasal pyramid secondary to a nasal fracture. Nasal alignment after nasal trauma is best assessed from directly in front of the patient where even subtle changes can be recognised. This should be delayed to 5–7 days after the injury to allow swelling to go down.

bony and cartilaginous structures should be palpated both externally and internally for crepitus and dislocation, which indicate a fracture.

Signs of severe fractures include lid oedema, periorbital ecchymosis, subconjunctival haemorrhage and subcutaneous emphysema. Care should also be taken to look for associated injuries such as cervical spine injury, mandibular fractures, orbital fractures (look for paraesthesia, step deformity, diplopia, epiphora, and evaluate eye movements for symmetry) and zygomatic fractures.

Investigation

When an uncomplicated nasal fracture is suspected, plain radiography is not indicated because of its poor sensitivity and specificity. However, some centres continue to advocate nasal films for legal documentation purposes. For more severe trauma, such as naso-orbital fractures, nasofrontal ethmoid fractures or possible cribriform plate fractures, CT scans should be obtained.

Management

Accurate, timely diagnosis and appropriate surgical treatment are important in the management of nasal fractures. After ensuring airway patency, adequate ventilation and the overall stability of the patient, treatment begins with management of external soft tissue injuries. It is critical to rule out septal haematomas. They may appear as a soft to firm swelling on one or both sides of the septum, and if present should be drained immediately. Failure to identify and treat a septal haematoma can result in a saddle deformity of the septum, which will require surgical repair.

Management of acute nasal fractures is confined largely to closed reduction of mild unilateral fractures under general anaesthetic. The goal is to realign cartilaginous and bony structures to their preinjury locations to maximise airway patency. The aesthetic outcomes of closed reduction are often less than optimal, and patients should be counselled that nasal reconstruction (septorhinoplasty) might eventually be necessary. Reduction should be done 5–10 days after the injury up to 2 weeks, and before the nasal bones start to fixate. Manual realignment (with or without instrumentation) is the easiest method of closed reduction.

Prognosis

Patients should expect to make a good recovery with acceptable cosmetic appearance and adequate nasal patency, but they should be warned that injuries may alter the anatomy of the nose.

Clinical insight

Nasal fractures are optimally dealt with 7–10 days after injury once the swelling has settled and before the bony fragments have fixed. In patients presenting much later a formal septorhinoplasty is usually required to achieve a good functional and cosmetic result.

Complications

Complications include:
- Cosmetic deformity
- Airway obstruction

- Haematoma
- Continuing epistaxis
- Rarely CSF rhinorrhoea.

4.7 Granulomatous conditions of the nose and paranasal sinuses

These are a group of disorders characterised by chronic inflammation and granuloma formation, which consists of monocytes, macrophages and epithelioid giant cells. They can easily be missed if not considered, which can have an impact on treatment and even survival in severe cases.

Epidemiology

These conditions are uncommon. The reported incidence varies, especially with respect to nasal and sinus involvement.

- **Wegener's granulomatosis** has an annual incidence of 5–9 per million of the adult population in Europe, where the age of presentation ranges from 15 to 65 and the male:female ratio is 1:1.
- **Sarcoidosis** has an annual incidence of 70–640 per million adults in Europe. It usually presents between 30 and 50 years of age, with a male:female ratio of 1:2. It is approximately three times more common in people of African descent than Caucasians.

Causes and pathogenesis

These can be infective, traumatic, inflammatory or neoplastic. Some of the causes are listed in **Table 4.7**, but the focus here is on the two most common inflammatory conditions, Wegener's granulomatosis and sarcoidosis.

The precise aetiology of Wegener's granulomatosis is not known. Cytoplasmic antineutrophil cytoplasmic antibodies (C-ANCA) are highly associated with disease activity.

Sarcoidosis is thought to be due to an imbalance between humoral and cell-mediated immunity triggered by stimulation of an antigen-presenting cell attracting macrophages into the region to form a granuloma similar to that of TB, but with no caseation.

Causes of granulomatous conditions	
Infective Bacterial	Tuberculosis and atypical mycobacteria Syphilis Actinomycosis Rhinoscleroma Leprosy
Fungal	Aspergillus Phyco- or mucormycosis Rhinosporidiosis Histoplasmosis
Parasitic	Leishmaniasis Toxoplasmosis
Traumatic	Pyogenic granuloma Foreign body granuloma
Inflammatory	Wegener's granulomatosis Sarcoidosis Cholesterol granuloma Eosinophilic granuloma Churg–Strauss syndrome
Neoplastic	T-cell lymphoma

Table 4.7 Causes of granulomatous conditions of the nose and paranasal sinuses

Clinical features

Wegener's granulomatosis

The nose (**Figure 4.7**) and paranasal sinuses are the most commonly involved organs, but any part of the body can be affected, mainly the lungs. It can start simply with nasal congestion, crusting, epistaxis or facial pain. If untreated, it progresses rapidly to involve other parts, and can be fatal. The symptoms depend on the organ involved, but the patient is generally unwell and pyrexial, with weight loss. Nasal examination reveals thickened mucosa, ulceration, crusting, septal perforation or nasal collapse.

Sarcoidosis

This is also a multisystem disease that can affect many parts of the body but often has ENT manifestations. A 'strawberry

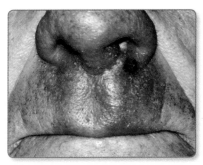

Figure 4.7 Wegner's granulomatosis affecting the nose and surrounding area. The dye marks the area where the skin biopsy was taken.

skin' appearance of the nasal mucosa has been described and congestion, crusting and bleeding are common. A purulent discharge is a feature of secondary infection. A mass can be seen externally when the disease penetrates and destroys the nasal bones (lupus pernio).

> **Clinical insight**
>
> Nasal crusting, especially with bloodstained discharge, should alert one to the possibility of granulomatous inflammation and prompt appropriate investigations.

Investigation

The key is to have a low level of suspicion and question generalised symptoms.

- **Blood tests** include FBC, urea and electrolytes, liver function tests, erythrocyte sedimentation rate, C-reactive protein, c-ANCA for Wegener's granulomatosis and serum ACE levels for sarcoidosis
- **Culture and sensitivity** when infective causes are suspected
- **Chest X-ray** and lung function test for pulmonary involvement
- **Urinalysis** for renal involvement
- **Biopsy** taken from affected nasal mucosa shows non-caseating granulomatous inflammation
- **Cross-sectional imaging** is useful in assessing the extent of the disease and for surgical planning.

Management

Management is multidisciplinary, involving the relevant medical specialties.

- Rheumatologists treat the inflammatory conditions with a mixture of steroids and various immune-modulating agents
- Antimicrobials are used to treat the infective causes and secondary infections
- Symptomatic treatment of nasal symptoms, especially crusting, includes saline douches, topical creams and steroids
- Surgery is generally to be avoided in active Wegener's granulomatosis and sarcoidosis, except for taking biopsies or decrusting, but is effective in foreign body, pyogenic and cholesterol granulomas.

> **Clinical insight**
>
> Granulomatous conditions affecting the nose can be locally destructive leading to nasal collapse and septal perforation. Rhinoplasty surgery for nasal augmentation or closure of a septal perforation should not be considered until the disease has remained inactive for several years.

Prognosis

Patients with Wegener's granulomatosis and sarcoidosis will require lifelong treatment, with considerable side effects or relapses. Kidney, eye, CNS and heart involvement carries a poor prognosis. Neoplastic aetiologies require radical treatment, and the prognosis depends highly on the stage at presentation. Infective and traumatic causes in general carry a better outcome.

4.8 Sinonasal tumours

These are benign or malignant neoplasms of the nose and sinuses. They may be epithelial or non-epithelial in origin.

Epidemiology

Malignant sinonasal tumours are rare and comprise less than 10% of head and neck cancers. The incidence is less than 1 in

100 000. In males it is double that in females, and patients often present in the fifth decade of life. Fifty per cent of nasal cavity tumours are benign and 50% are malignant. The majority of paranasal sinus tumours are malignant.

Causes and pathogenesis

The sinonasal region exhibits a wide diversity of tumour subtypes compared to other regions in the body (**Table 4.8**). Adenocarcinoma of the ethmoid sinuses is related to the hardwood industry and leather tanning chemicals. Other carcinogenic agents implicated include nickel refining fumes, mineral oils, radium, lacquer paint, chromium and cigarette smoking. Epstein–Barr virus may be responsible in the aetiology of nasopharyngeal malignancy. Dietary factors have been implicated in the high prevalence of nasopharyngeal malignancies in southern China.

Clinical features

Sinonasal tumours present with nasal blockage (especially unilateral), epistaxis, anosmia, pain and nasal discharge. Diplopia is a serious feature suggesting orbital involvement.

Epithelial	Nonepithelial	Lymphoreticular tumors
Squamous cell carcinoma (SCC) Transitional cell carcinoma (TCC) Adenocarcinoma Adenoid cystic carcinoma Melanoma Olfactory neuroblastoma Undifferentiated carcinoma	Soft-tissue sarcoma Rhabdomyosarcoma Leiomyosarcoma Fibrosarcoma Liposarcoma Angiosarcoma Myxosarcoma Hemangiopericytoma Connective tissue sarcoma Chondrosarcoma Osteosarcoma Synovial sarcoma	Lymphoma Plasmacytoma Giant cell tumor Metastatic carcinoma

Table 4.8 Wide diversity of tumour subtypes exhibited in the sinonasal region

A full examination is necessary, including the face, oral cavity, and oropharynx, with anterior rhinoscopy, neck examination and examination of the nasal cavity with a flexible nasendoscope or rigid Hopkins rod telescope. Particular attention is paid to unilateral nasal polypi/masses. It is necessary to assess and document their size, surface, colour and position in the nose.

Investigation

Plain radiography has been superseded by **CT scans** of the nose and paranasal sinuses. These can be particularly valuable in suspected malignancy when combined with MRI, as this helps differentiate fluid from solid matter (**Figure 4.8**). All unilateral masses in the nose and sinuses must be **biopsied** and assessed by examination under anaesthesia, or by endoscopic sinus surgery for histology if the sinuses are involved.

Management

Management depends on the histology of the tumour.

Inverted papilloma

This must be completely removed, either via endoscopic excision, lateral rhinotomy or midfacial degloving. An incomplete

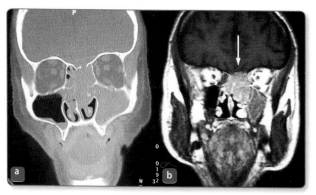

Figure 4.8 Left-sided sinonasal malignancy. (a) CT and (b) MRI.

excision results in recurrence (15–78% depending on method of excision) and careful endoscopic follow-up is necessary to check for recurrence. Malignant change can occur (2–27%), with squamous cell carcinoma the commonest.

Juvenile angiofibroma

Juvenile angiofibroma is a purple vascular mass occuring almost exclusively in teenage boys. It arises from the sphenopalatine foramen, and therefore originates from the nasal cavity rather than the nasopharynx which it grows to occupy. Preoperative embolisation may be helpful prior to complete surgical excision usually by a midfacial degloving approach, which avoids a facial scar.

Cancer of the maxillary antrum

This often presents late. A bloodstained nasal discharge and unilateral nasal obstruction may be the early features. Swelling of the cheek, bleeding or ulceration of the gum and palate, referred pain to the ear, head or jaw, epiphora, proptosis and double vision denote involvement of the surrounding structures and are late presenting features.

Depending on their location, most malignancies require resection followed by postoperative radiotherapy. Operations include:

- Medial maxillectomy
- Inferior maxillectomy
- Total maxillectomy
- Radical maxillectomy
- Craniofacial resection and anterior skull base surgery allows for excision of the sinonasal tumour together with the cribriform plate and anterior cranial fossa tumour extension. Neck dissection to deal with the lymph nodes may also be necessary.

Nasopharyngeal malignancies

These also present late with nasal obstruction and a bloodstained nasal discharge. Unilateral otitis media resulting in conductive hearing loss due to blockage of the Eustachian tube is also a late sign. Extension laterally to the parapharyngeal space can cause facial, palatal and pharyngeal loss of sensation with involvement of the trigeminal nerve (V), and trismus with pterygoid muscle involvement. Spread into the retrostyloid space involves the cervical sympathetics and cranial nerves IX, X, XI, XII with resultant Horner's syndrome, hoarseness, dysphagia, shoulder weakness and tongue weakness. Superior spread to the foramen lacerum involves cranial nerves III, IV and V causing diplopia, facial numbness and headaches.

Clinical insight

Unilateral hearing loss with nasal obstruction and a bloodstained discharge is an ominous sign. It must arouse suspicion and the nasopharynx needs to be examined by an otolaryngologist. Sinonasal tumours, including nasopharyngeal carcinomas, often present late, with nodal spread and involvement of surrounding structures.

Treatment of a small nasopharyngeal carcinoma may be solely by radiotherapy. Larger tumours may require additional chemotherapy. Surgery is rarely used although may be adopted to deal with neck node metastases or after failed radiotherapy.

Head and neck

Most head and neck presentations with recent-onset hoarseness, difficulty in swallowing or a lump in the neck require an urgent (2 weeks) referral. Airway compromise secondary to head and neck pathology may present as an emergency.

5.1 Clinical scenarios

Hoarseness (dysphonia)

Background

A 58-year-old lecturer attended his GP with a 2-week history of hoarseness following a lower respiratory tract infection. On closer questioning it became clear that his voice had progressively worsened over 3 months and become quite 'deep and gravelly'. He also had noticed intermittent bloodstained phlegm. On subsequent referral to ENT via the 2-week suspected cancer pathway, there are no other upper aerodigestive symptoms such as dysphagia, odynophagia, stridor, neck swelling or referred otalgia.

History

The patient is otherwise fit and healthy, with mild chronic obstructive airway disease. He has smoked 15–20 cigarettes per day for the last 30 years, and consumes 20–30 units of alcohol per week. He is taking omeprazole 20 mg once daily for long-standing dyspepsia.

Examination

A full ENT examination, including otoscopy, oral cavity and flexible nasendoscopy (nasopharyngoscopy), reveal a warty white lesion over the anterior one third of the right true vocal fold. There is full movement (abduction and adduction) of the vocal folds. Palpation of the neck does not reveal any lymphadenopathy.

Investigation

A CT scan of the neck is performed prior to biopsy to determine the extent of the tumour, airway patency, cartilage involvement, subglottic extent and potential involvement of the paraglottic space and lymph nodes. Blood tests are performed to evaluate anaemia, nutrition and electrolytes.

Under general anaesthesia, a microlaryngoscopy is performed to examine the supraglottis (aryepiglottic folds, arytenoids and false vocal folds), the glottis (true vocal folds) and the subglottis (lower border of glottis to cricoid) (**Figure 5.1**). An excisional biopsy is performed.

All the investigations are discussed at the local multidisciplinary team (MDT) meeting.

> **Clinical insight**
>
> Presentation with recent onset hoarseness (more than 4 weeks duration), difficulty in swallowing, or a lump in the neck requires an urgent referral (within 2 weeks).

Differential diagnosis

Table 5.1 shows the main differentials of a patient presenting with hoarseness.

- **Malignant tumours of the larynx** A short history of persistent hoarseness with no improvement with conservative measures should arouse suspicion of a malignant glottal lesion
- **Precancerous lesions:** the presentation is similar to malignant lesion

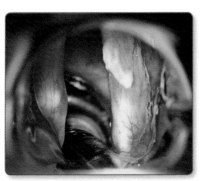

Figure 5.1
Microlaryngoscopy findings of a lesion of the right vocal fold in a smoker who presented with hoarseness.

Type of lesion	Possible diagnosis
Malignant tumours of the larynx	Carcinoma *in situ* Squamous cell carcinoma Undifferentiated carcinoma Adenocarcinoma Adenoid cystic and chondrosarcoma
Precancerous lesions	Erythroplakia Leukoplakia
Benign lesions	Vocal nodules Vocal cysts and polyps, Reinke's oedema Laryngeal papilloma
Inflammatory lesions	Chronic granulomatous conditions, e.g. Wegener's granulomatosis Sarcoidosis
Infective conditions	Fungal infections (*Candida*) Tuberculosis

Table 5.1 Conditions associated with hoarseness and possible diagnoses

- **Benign lesions:** these benign lesions have often a longer duration of dysphonia, and have characteristic features on laryngoscopic assessment (see section 5.3)
- **Chronic inflammatory conditions:** the history in Wegener's granulomatosis and sarcoidosis is often longer than other presentations
- **Infective conditions:** fungal infections (e.g. *Candida*) can be seen in asthmatics who use steroid inhalers without a spacer device. Infection may not be limited to the glottis and could affect surrounding areas (e.g. supraglottis)
- **Tuberculosis:** isolated laryngeal tuberculosis is uncommon; it often involves the chest and the classic features of pulmonary tuberculosis (cough, night sweats, weight loss) may also be present.

Discussion

The diagnosis here is squamous cell carcinoma of the glottis. Glottal lesions present early, as hoarseness is an early symptom. The reduced lymphatics at glottal level are an impediment to rapid spread into the lymph nodes. However, supraglottic and hypopharyngeal lesions present with nodal spread early on owing to the rich supply of lymphatics. Glottal tumours, if picked up early without nodal involvement, have a much better prognosis.

> ## Clinical insight
>
> A smoker with a change in voice (hoarseness) and cough may not have another 'chest infection' – laryngeal assessment is essential. Hoarseness persisting for more than 4 weeks should be referred for laryngoscopy.

Dysphagia
Background
A 48-year-old woman had long-standing intermittent dysphagia which worsened over 6 weeks, first in relation to solids and then fluids. She had persistent pain in the throat and otalgia. Her swallowing gradually deteriorated and she was finding it difficult to complete a meal.

History
She has iron deficiency anaemia, for which she takes ferrous sulphate. She smokes 20 cigarettes per day but does not drink.

Examination
The patient is apyrexial. She looks cachectic and has been losing weight over a number of months. Her oral cavity, oropharynx, anterior rhinoscopy and neck examinations are normal. Nasendoscopy does not reveal any mucosal lesion, and both vocal cords are normal with normal mobility. However, pooling of saliva posterolateral to the arytenoids is seen in the pyriform fossae.

Investigation
The FBC shows iron deficiency anaemia. A barium swallow is ordered, which shows a stricture in the postcricoid area (**Figure 5.2**). To better visualise the postcricoid area, panendoscopy with or without biopsy would be needed.

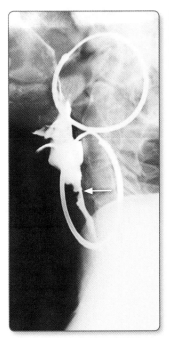

Figure 5.2 Barium swallow showing a filling defect (arrow) in the hypopharynx in a patient who presented with long-standing intermittent dysphagia.

Differential diagnosis

- **Postcricoid carcinoma** usually results in rapid progressive dysphagia associated with loss of weight and cachexia
- **Patterson–Kelly–Brown/Plummer–Vinson syndrome** consists of a triad of glossitis, iron deficiency anaemia and dysphagia which usually improves after iron replacement. The dysphagia is due to oesophageal web. It has been associated with increased risk of upper alimentary tract cancers
- **Benign oesophageal strictures** usually produce dysphagia with slow and insidious progression (i.e. months to years) of frequency and severity, with minimal weight loss

- **Achalasia or collagen vascular disorders** (motility disorders) cause dysphagia to solids and liquids simultaneously
- **Postcricoid web** usually has slower progression of dysphagia and rarely causes absolute dysphagia in the way that a neoplastic lesion does
- **Pharyngeal pouch** may manifest with regurgitation of undigested food and occasional gurgling
- **Globus pharyngeus** is usually intermittent and more often a 'feeling of a lump' in the throat rather than a true lump.

Discussion

The diagnosis here is a malignant stricture of the upper oesophagus. Malignant oesophageal strictures result in a rapid progression (i.e. weeks to months) of severity and frequency of dysphagia, and are frequently associated with significant weight loss. Prognosis and survival are poor compared with laryngeal cancers. When diagnosed early without regional, nodal or metastatic spread, treatment of malignant stricture is surgical (oesophagectomy). Sometimes chemotherapy, radiation, or a combination of the two may be used instead. Palliative treatment includes endoscopic dilation of the oesophagus, sometimes with placement of a stent to keep the oesophagus dilated.

> **Clinical insight**
>
> True dysphagia needs to be referred urgently (within 2 weeks). Barium swallow and pharyngoscopy/oesophagoscopy and upper GI endoscopy are essential to establish a diagnosis.

Neck lump

Background

A 32-year-old woman with no previous medical history presented to her GP with a neck swelling that had gradually increased in size over several months. She had no upper respiratory tract infection and was generally asymptomatic, but had recently felt pressure in and around the region of the lump. Despite having a normal FBC, she was treated with antibiotics (amoxicillin 125 mg three times daily for 5 days). However, the lump continued to grow very slowly and was also noted to regress spontaneously. Her GP was uncertain as to what the lump could be and sent her to the emergency department for further management.

History

The patient recently started to smoke. She drinks less than 10 units of alcohol per week. She has a cat at home.

Examination

After examining the patient, the triage nurse refers her to the resident ENT doctor, who finds nothing untoward on head and neck examination, except for a 4 x 3 cm fluctuant non-tender swelling in the left anterior triangle of the neck, below the angle of the mandible and in front of the sternocleidomastoid muscle (**Figure 5.3**).

> ### Clinical insight
>
> Cat scratch disease (*Bartonella henselae*) and toxoplasmosis (*Toxoplasma gondii*) should be considered in cases of lymphadenitis, especially when there has been close contact with cats. Relevant serological tests should be performed.

Investigation

A straw-coloured fluid is aspirated from the lump and sent for cytological/histopathological studies and microbiology (**Figure 5.4**). No conclusive results are noted besides some

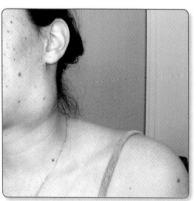

Figure 5.3 Cystic lump in the left anterior triangle of the neck.

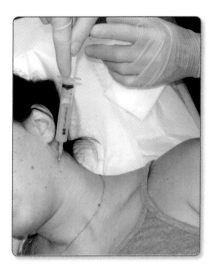

Figure 5.4 Fine-needle aspiration from a cystic neck lump for cytology.

macrophages and lymphocytes. All blood tests performed at this time are normal.

Differential diagnosis

- **Lateral cervical (branchial) cyst** usually presents as a painless, fluctuant mass in the anterior triangle of the neck. Lateral cervical cysts can rarely be cystic metastatic lymph nodes and a high index of suspicion is needed in smokers or those over 40 years of age.
- **Thyroglossal cyst** usually presents as a midline, painless spherical neck swelling which rises on tongue protrusion.
- **Submandibular gland hypertrophy, sialadenitis or sialolithiasis** will present as a neck swelling, but in level I of the neck below the ramus of the mandible.
- **Lymphadenitis** is associated with a tender neck swelling which may develop into a fluctuant neck abscess with overlying inflammatory skin changes.
- **Necrotic lymph node** secondary to TB or other granulomatous disease may present with a fluctuant 'cold' neck abscess.
- **Metastatic lymph node** has the possibility of presenting as a cystic neck mass.

- **Lymphovascular malformation** is due to malformed vessels of either the lymphatic or the vascular systems.
- **Paraganglioma** (e.g. carotid body tumour) presents as a pulsatile neck mass.

> ### Clinical insight
>
> - In the presence of a neck mass it is essential to examine the head and neck thoroughly, including the oral cavity and scalp, as well as performing a fibreoptic flexible nasendoscopy to exclude a potential primary site for malignancy
> - The first-line investigation is an ultrasound scan with fine-needle aspiration for cytology.

Discussion

The diagnosis here is a branchial cyst. Management is total excision under general anaesthesia via a transverse skin crease neck incision.

Airway compromise in an adult

Background

A 76-year-old Caucasian man who was recently discharged from the intensive care unit after an infective exacerbation of chronic bronchitis presents to the emergency department with worsening breathing difficulties. Over the past week he had consulted his GP and described increasing hoarseness, heartburn and an unproductive cough.

On chest examination there were no crepitations. He was treated with proton pump inhibitors for presumed reflux.

> ### Clinical insight
>
> Airway obstruction should be treated early, with the most senior ENT surgeon and anaesthetist involved.

History

There is a history of hypertension, hiatus hernia and chronic obstructive airways disease. The patient is a retired electrician who lives with his wife. He smokes 20 roll-up cigarettes a day and drinks 20 units of alcohol per week. He regularly takes bendroflumethiazide 2.5 mg daily, and becotide and salbutamol inhalers.

Examination

On presentation to the emergency department the patient has an inspiratory stridor (upper airway noises), is using his accessory muscles of respiration, and is unable to complete sentences. Examination of the nose, oral cavity, oropharynx and neck is unremarkable. Flexible fibreoptic nasendoscopy show an obstructive lesion of the larynx.

Investigation

Full blood count (FBC) confirms a microcytic anaemia but normal white blood cell count (WBC), urea and electrolytes reveal mild dehydration, and lung function tests and C-reactive protein (CRP) are normal. After initial treatment with an adrenaline nebuliser and intravenous steroid, the patient's condition improves slightly. The on-call anaesthetist is paged and an urgent panendoscopy organised. Microlaryngoscopy is carried out to further assess the larynx and take a biopsy (**Figure 5.5**).

Differential diagnosis

For acute stridor, the differentials are:

- **Infections** in the head and neck (e.g. epiglottitis, laryngitis, Ludwig's angina) with associated inflammatory swelling can cause significant airway compromise
- **Airway trauma** can lead to haematoma and oedema with airway compromise.
- **Anaphylaxis** causes rapid-onset airway obstruction
- **Foreign body,** such as a denture in an edentulous patient, may obstruct the airway
- **Postoperative haematoma**

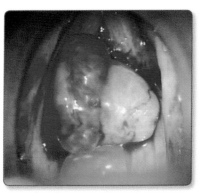

Figure 5.5 Endoscopic view showing an obstructing lesion arising from the left posterior glottis.

- **Bilateral vocal fold palsy** after surgery (e.g. total thyroidectomy) or rarely endotracheal intubation.

For chronic stridor, the differentials are:

- **Tumour** (e.g. laryngeal, thyroid, pharyngeal or mediastinal) can cause increasing airway obstruction with growth
- **Cricoarytenoid ankylosis** in rheumatoid arthritis will give rise to fixation of the vocal folds, limiting the glottic airway
- **Laryngeal inflammation** (e.g. Wegener's granulomatosis) is a rare cause of airway compromise
- **Arytenoid granuloma** can develop after intubation, with a fleshy mass in the posterior larynx.

Discussion

The diagnosis here is squamous cell carcinoma of the larynx. Management involves discussion at the multidisciplinary cancer team meeting and a review of imaging and histology. Appropriate treatment depends on the TNM stage of the tumour (see pp. 177 and 193).

Airway obstruction should be treated early by an expert team. The severity (mild, moderate, severe) and level of obstruction guide immediate treatment. In general, the least invasive method that will bypass the obstruction should be used.

> ### Clinical insight
>
> Following prolonged endotracheal intubation there is a possibility of laryngeal trauma resulting in a granuloma. This is often worsened with reflux and coughing.

5.2 Tonsillitis and peritonsillar abscess (quinsy)

Tonsillitis is inflammation due to infection of the palatine tonsils, lymphoid tissue found in the lateral wall of the oropharynx. The inflammation can often spread to the associated lingual tonsils adjacent to the tongue base and the pharyngeal tonsils (adenoids) in the nasopharynx. It may spread laterally beyond the palatine tonsils, causing peritonsillar cellulitis, which may lead to the formation of a peritonsillar abscess, also termed quinsy.

Epidemiology

Tonsillitis can affect anyone but most commonly occurs in children, although rarely under the age of 2. Bacterial tonsillitis commonly affects children aged 5–15 years, whereas viral tonsillitis is more common at a younger age. Peritonsillar abscess tends to occur in teens or young adults, but may present earlier.

A family history of atopy and of tonsillectomy may predict the occurrence of tonsillitis in an individual.

Causes

Most cases of tonsillitis are viral; 15–30% are caused by bacteria.

The common cold viruses, including adenovirus, rhinovirus, coronavirus and RSV (respiratory syncytial virus) are the most common viral causes. Others viruses implicated include EBV (Epstein–Barr virus – infectious mononucleosis), herpes simplex, cytomegalovirus, measles and HIV.

Group A beta-haemolytic *Streptococcus pyogenes* causes most bacterial tonsillitis. *Staphylococcus aureus*, *Streptococcus pneumoniae*, and *Haemophilus influenzae* are also often isolated in recurrent tonsillitis. Rarer causes include *Mycoplasma pneumoniae*, *Chlamydia pneumoniae*, *Bordetella pertussis*, *Corynebacterium diphtheriae*, syphilis and gonorrhoea. Anaerobes including *Bacteroides* spp. play a role in chronic tonsillitis. A polymicrobial flora is isolated from peritonsillar abscesses.

Other factors contributing to the development of tonsillitis include immunodeficiency, overcrowding, malnourishment and radiation exposure.

Pathogenesis

The viral incubation period is usually 2–4 days. Tonsillitis can spread from person to person through hand-to-mouth contact, via airborne droplets, or by sharing the utensils or toothbrush of an infected person.

Clinical features

Symptoms include fever, sore throat, halitosis, dysphagia (difficulty swallowing), odynophagia (painful swallowing), headache, referred otalgia, lethargy and malaise. Younger children may complain of abdominal pain and vomiting. Airway obstruction may manifest as mouth breathing, snoring, nocturnal breathing pauses, or sleep apnoea.

Symptoms usually resolve in 3–4 days but may last up to 2 weeks despite adequate therapy.

Signs include:

- Erythema and enlargement of the tonsils, which may be covered in exudates (see **Figure 6.3**). Infectious mononucleosis (EBV) can exhibit profuse exudates on the tonsils (**Figure 5.6**). Patients may also have splenomegaly and axillary or inguinal lymphadenopathy
- Tender and enlarged cervical lymph nodes
- Skin rash: scarlet fever, which is rare, is caused by an exotoxin released by *Streptococcus pyogenes*. The condition is characterised by a punctate erythematous rash (**Figure 5.7**), whiteness around the mouth, and a 'strawberry and cream' tongue.

Recurrent tonsillitis (warranting tonsillectomy) This is defined as seven episodes in 1 year, five infections in 2 consecutive years, or three infections each year for 3 consecutive years.

Chronic tonsillitis   This manifests as chronic sore throat, halitosis, tonsillitis, and persistent tender cervical nodes.

Peritonsillar cellulitis/abscess   Symptoms include severe sore throat (usually worse one side) fever, drooling, trismus (difficulty opening the mouth due to inflammation spread to the pterygoid

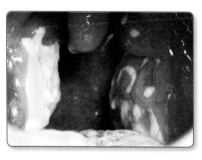

Figure 5.6 Glandular fever with exudates.

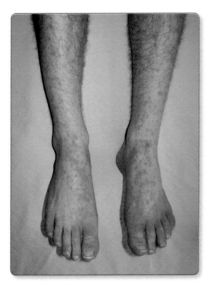

Figure 5.7 Classic skin rash manifested by a streptococcal sore throat

muscles), halitosis and altered voice quality (the 'hot potato' voice). Unilateral bulging of the mucosa above and lateral to the tonsils is pathognomonic.

Investigation
- Blood tests including FBC (raised WBC), urea and electrolytes (dehydration), CRP (raised), ESR (raised), and Epstein Barr virus serology (for glandular fever)
- Pus aspirated from a peritonsillar abscess should be sent for microscopy, culture and sensitivity studies
- Throat swabs may be taken from high-risk (e.g. immuno-compromised) patients and those for whom treatment fails.

Diagnosis
The Centor criteria (**Table 5.2**) are used to aid the diagnosis of tonsillitis caused by bacteria (group A beta-hemolytic strep-tococci (GABHS), in particular). If a patient has 3 or 4 of the criteria, it is likely there is a bacterial infection. The absence of

Centor criteria	Significance of score
Each of following scores 1 point: • History of fever • Tonsillar exudates • Absence of cough • Tender cervical lympadenopathy	0–1: Unlikely to have GABHS. Likely viral sore throat which should be treated symptomatically with analgesia and fluids 2: Possible GABHS, treat as above initially. Consider antibiotics after 48–72 hours if worsening symptoms. It is not routine practice to take a throat swab, unless clinical concern, e.g. immunocompromised, recent travel abroad 3–4: Consider starting antibiotic as 40–60% chance of GABHS

Table 5.2 Centor criteria to aid diagnosis of group A beta-haemolytic streptoccocal sore throat

3 or 4 means it is unlikely bacterial and is associated with an 80% negative predictive value.

Tonsillar size is normally graded using the Brodsky classification:
• Grade I – tonsils within the tonsillar fossa
• Grade II – tonsils protruding to the level of the anterior tonsillar pillar
• Grade III – tonsils causing a 50–75% obstruction of the airway
• Grade IV – tonsils causing >75% airway obstruction (often touching – i.e. 'kissing' tonsils) (see **Figure 6.3**).

Management

Patients with tonsillitis who are able to eat and drink may be discharged home with oral antibiotics, analgesia and rehydration. However, patients who are unable to drink due to acute swelling of the tonsils, as well as those with a peritonsillar abscess, should be treated as an inpatient with intravenous antibiotics and fluids and parenteral analgesia, until they are able to recommence oral intake.

IV corticosteroids may be given in the first 24 hours to reduce tonsillar swelling. On discharge IV antibiotics can be changed to oral to complete a total course of 7–10 days, and appropriate analgesia given which may need to be soluble medication. Typical combination broad-spectrum antibiotic therapy would be benzylpenicillin (IV) or phenoxymethylpenicillin (PO) and metronidazole – these may vary according to local prescribing guidelines. Amoxicillin and ampicillin compounds should be avoided as they can cause a generalised papular rash in infectious mononucleosis. Clarithromycin may be used in cases of penicillin allergy.

If there is clinical suspicion of a peritonsillar abscess, needle aspiration (with a 19G needle) into the most prominent area of the peritonsillar bulge or incision and drainage using a no 15 blade scalpel should be performed after the application of topical local anaesthetic spray. Drainage of pus will often bring about swift relief of pain.

Adequate rest for patients with tonsillitis accelerates recovery. Patients diagnosed with infectious mononucleosis must be cautioned against activities that may cause abdominal injury, as this may lead to splenic rupture.

Infection may be prevented by avoiding contact with individuals who are ill or patients who are immunocompromised. Some research supports the use of the antipneumococcal vaccine to prevent acute tonsillitis.

Patients with a history of recurrent tonsillitis (see p. 163) or peritonsillar abscess may be considered for interval tonsillectomy. This is best performed when the tonsils are not acutely inflamed, as otherwise the risk of perioperative bleeding is higher. In April 2010 the Scottish Intercollegiate Guidelines Network (SIGN) published updated guidelines entitled *Management of sore throat and indications for tonsillectomy*, available at www.sign.ac.uk.

Prognosis and complications

Untreated or incompletely treated tonsillitis can lead to potentially life-threatening complications:

- Infection may spread from a peritonsillar abscess to the adjacent parapharyngeal or retropharyngeal deep neck

spaces. Further progression can lead to mediastinitis or even necrotising fasciitis
- Rarely, acute tonsillitis may lead to thrombophlebitis of the internal jugular vein
- Complications specific to GABHS pharyngitis are scarlet fever, rheumatic fever, septic arthritis and glomerulonephritis.

5.3 Globus pharyngeus

Globus pharyngeus is a feeling of a lump or irritation in the throat in the absence of a physical abnormality.

Epidemiology

Globus affects up to 35% of men and 50% of women. It accounts for 3–4% of ENT outpatient referrals.

Causes and pathogenesis

Globus pharyngeus is often precipitated by a significant adverse personal event. A variety of causes have been implicated:
- Gastro-oesophageal reflux
- Laryngopharyngeal reflux (**Figure 5.8**)
- Cricopharyngeal spasm

> **Clinical insight**
>
> Reflux is a common cause of globus pharyngeus and is easily treatable for cough and hoarseness.

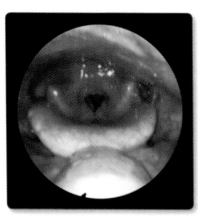

Figure 5.8 Flexible laryngoscopy showing redness and oedema of the posterior larynx, suggesting laryngopharyngeal reflux.

- Tonsillar hypertrophy
- Thyroid lumps
- Cervical osteophytes.

Clinical features

The patient feels an irritation or lump in the throat which is either intermittent or continuous. They have no sinister symptoms of pain in the throat, otalgia, hoarseness of voice, dysphagia or weight loss. It is often worse in the morning and improves with oral intake. It may be exacerbated by the consumption of acidic drinks, or spicy or salty foods that dry the throat. It is often associated with frequent throat clearing and dry cough, which serve to dry the throat further and exacerbate the problem.

Investigation

Complete examination of the oral cavity, oropharynx, anterior rhinoscopy, neck, and **nasendoscopy** of the larynx and pharynx. Normally the physical examination is unremarkable, or there may be some erythema of the arytenoids and posterior laryngopharynx suggestive of reflux disease.

> ### Clinical insight
> The absence of heartburn does not rule out laryngopharyngeal reflux, as 50% of patients with laryngopharyngeal reflux do not experience overt heartburn.

Diagnosis

The diagnosis is based on the history and an unremarkable physical examination. With an appropriate clinical picture and in the absence of dysphagia or food sticking, further investigations are not usually required. However, in the presence of such symptoms a barium swallow may sometimes be required to rule out any lesion of the hypopharynx/upper oesophagus, or where there is a high level of anxiety, to help reassure the patient. In some units flexible transnasal fibreoptic oesophagoscopy can be offered in the outpatient setting to inspect the hypopharynx and oesophagus directly.

Management

Management includes advice and medical treatment. Advice for patients with globus pharyngeus is:

- Strong reassurance that there is nothing sinister
- Sip water regularly to improve hydration
- Avoid chronic throat clearing and coughing
- Avoid spicy and salty foods
- Avoid acidic drinks
- Avoid smoking and excess alcohol. Medically, an empirical 6-week course of a proton pump inhibitor can be helpful, especially where there is evidence of posterior laryngitis and laryngopharyngeal reflux. The patient should be reviewed after this treatment and, if still symptomatic, endoscopy considered, which could be either a direct rigid panendoscopy under general anaesthesia or a flexible oesophagoscopy (either transnasal or transoral).

Prognosis

The majority of patients improve with the above conservative and medical measures. If they do not respond to treatment it is most commonly due to persistent throat clearing, which they have not managed to suppress adequately.

5.4 Voice disorders and vocal fold pathology

Vocal fold lesions, which encompass several distinct pathological entities, are a common cause of hoarseness (dysphonia).

Epidemiology

The annual incidence of voice disorders varies from 28 to 121/100 000.

Causes

The causes of voice disorders are listed in **Table 5.3**.

Investigation

Vocal disorders range from complete absence of the voice (aphonia) to varying degrees of vocal impairment (dysphonia). Ideally, patients with voice disorders should be seen in a multidisciplinary voice clinic, with the laryngologist and speech and language therapist working as a co-ordinated team.

History and assessment

Patients will usually describe how their voice sounds and any associated discomfort at rest and during phonation. A detailed history must be taken to include initial upper respiratory tract infection/laryngitis, voice use/misuse/abuse, laryngopharyngeal reflux, occupation, smoking, alcohol, history of intubation, stridor. Information is obtained on the patient's lifestyle, health, social history, and occupation and stress factors. Listen to the patient's voice and observe their vocal and non-vocal behaviour.

Infective	Acute/chronic laryngitis
Inflammatory	Reinke's oedema (**Figure 5.10**) Granulomatous disorders
Structural	Vocal fold nodules Vocal fold polyp Vocal cysts and sulci
Neurological	Vocal fold paralysis
Traumatic	Internal: contact ulcer & granuloma Surgical (thyroid, neck, mediastinal, cardiac surgery) Non-surgical (blunt and penetrating trauma)
Neoplastic	Benign tumours (laryngeal papillomatosis, chondroma) Malignant tumours (squamous cell carcinoma)
Miscellaneous	Endocrine (hypothyroid) Autoimmune conditions

Table 5.3 Causes of voice disorders

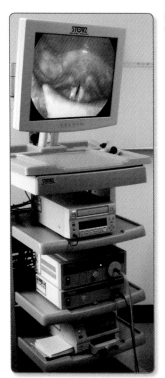

Figure 5.9 Video endoscopic system for evaluation of the larynx.

Laryngeal evaluation

This provides information about laryngeal structure and function. Techniques, such as video **laryngo-stroboscopy (Figure 5.9)** which involves video recording laryngeal movements with special stroboscopic light, can provide accessible information and documentation.

Perceptual evaluation

Acoustic profile – instrumental analysis of the voice gives baseline measures to monitor the progress of treatment. Abnormalities of the voice can involve one or more of the vocal parameters: pitch, pitch range, loudness, resonance, flexibility and stamina. A particular vocal profile is to be expected when the larynx has been visualised, e.g. with a unilateral mass lesion on the true vocal fold, the pitch is commonly lowered and there is roughness of the fundamental frequency.

Radiological and haematological investigations

Chest X-rays and CT scans tracing the recurrent laryngeal nerve (skull base to mediastinum) are the investigations of choice in vocal fold paralysis. CT and MRI now offer 3D reconstructed images of the larynx and virtual 'endoscopy'. Specific haematological tests, e.g. thyroid function tests, are also useful where hypothyroidism is suspected.

> ### Clinical insight
>
> Hoarseness and voice changes can be due to pathology elsewhere: you need to think 'outside the box'! (In particular, see discussion of vocal fold palsy on p. 174.)

Pathogenesis, clinical features and management

There are three general approaches to the management of voice problems: medical, surgical and behavioural, including speech therapy.

Vocal fold nodules (Singer's nodules)

These are bilateral mass lesions at the junction of the anterior one third and the posterior two thirds of the true vocal fold, creating an hourglass-shaped glottis chink. These arise from trauma to the mucosa due to hyperfunctional phonation. There is a gradual onset of dysphonia, initially episodic but eventually constant, with effortful phonation and vocal tract discomfort. The lesions are initially soft but can become fibrosed.

Speech therapy is the treatment of choice. Phonosurgery may be required for fibrosed nodules, but voice therapy is essential to change vocal behaviour and prevent recurrence.

Vocal fold polyp

This a unilateral sessile or pedunculated polyp, located usually on the free edge of the anterior vocal fold. It occurs as a result of acute trauma to the vocal fold mucosa combined with infection. It presents with dysphonia, vocal tract discomfort and a reported sensation of 'something' in the throat. A trial of speech therapy can be given initially for small sessile polyps, before considering phonosurgery. Larger sessile and pedunculated polyps require surgical excision, preceded and followed by speech therapy.

Contact ulcers

These occur on the posterior part of the vocal fold which overlies the vocal process of the arytenoid cartilage. They occur after hyperfunction phonation with a forced, effortful and low-pitched voice, in association with laryngopharyngeal reflux. There is a gradual onset of dysphonia, with marked vocal tract discomfort. Treatment is speech therapy for early lesions and anti-reflux treatment.

Reinke's oedema

This involves the superficial layer of the lamina propria, which fills and becomes oedematous over the superior surface of the vocal fold bilaterally (**Figure 5.10**). Prolonged smoking and

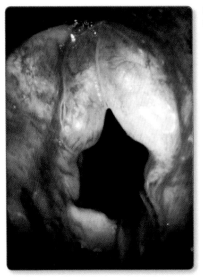

Figure 5.10 Reinke's oedema of the vocal folds.

vocal abuse are the primary causes, leading to low-pitched effortful phonation. Phonosurgery is the primary treatment in combination with pre- and postoperative speech therapy.

Vocal fold paralysis

This can be partial or complete; the vocal folds are unable to meet in the midline and a glottal gap results in a breathy or hoarse voice. The recurrent laryngeal nerve supplying the larynx can be affected in its long course from the skull base to the mediastinum. The left side is more commonly affected, as the left recurrent laryngeal nerve has a longer course (see p. 19). The nerve can be affected in the chest (carcinoma bronchus, malignant mediastinal nodes, aortic aneurysm, cardiac and oesophageal surgery, carcinoma oesophagus). It could also be injured in thyroid and other surgical procedures in the neck. Idiopathic and viral infections are other causes of vocal fold paralysis. Bilateral vocal fold palsy is a rare condition but may present dramatically with stridor following thyroid surgery, or with thyroid malignancy; treatment in the stridulous patient is urgent tracheostomy.

Treatment for unilateral vocal fold palsy is aimed at closing the glottal gap, especially where compensation is inadequate. Speech therapy aims at improving glottal closure, failing which surgery is planned. In patients with partial palsy or where the cause is idiopathic or viral, it is usually worth waiting 6 months for neural function to recover. Surgery is carried out with a view to medialising (bringing the affected fold closer to the midline), with either an internal injection or a silastic block placed as an implant through a cartilage window in the larynx (thyroplasty). Conservative vocal treatment measures include:

- Vocal hygiene (absolute silence and whispering not advised)
- Alter vocal behaviour
- Fluid hydration
- Cough suppression
- Proton pump inhibitors (twice-daily dosing for a minimum of 3 months)
- Lifestyle and dietary changes
- Stop smoking and reduce alcohol consumption.

5.5 Thyroid swelling

Common clinical thyroid swellings are cysts and nodules – solitary and multiple, inflammatory lesions (e.g. thyroiditis), and benign adenomas. Thyroid nodules are common. The majority of swellings are benign and 4–7% are malignant. There is a female preponderance. The risk of malignancy is greater with solitary nodules or in patients with risk factors, e.g. a family history of thyroid cancer, or radiation exposure. Most thyroid cancers are associated with a good prognosis if treated early.

Thyroid swellings can present as neck swellings or can be incidental findings, especially on ultrasound.

Epidemiology

Thyroid swellings affect 5% of the world population and are endemic in areas of iodine deficiency. The majority are due to thyroid hypofunction. A palpable thyroid (goitre) can be physiological if the patient is pregnant or going through puberty.

Pathogenesis

Thyroid swellings are slow growing. Hypo- or hyperfunction is usually associated with a benign pathology. Rapid growth suggests bleeding into the swelling/cyst, or malignancy. Associated pain may be indicative of inflammatory pathology, i.e. thyroiditis. Any associated dysphagia, dysphonia and/or stridor with thyroid swelling needs urgent investigation and management. Drugs such as lithium, amiodarone and antithyroid medication can induce goitre.

Clinical features

Most patients have a slow-growing swelling over a long period. The commonest presentation is a visible thyroid swelling (**Figure 5.11**). Other features include change in voice due to involvement of the recurrent laryngeal nerve; dysphagia may be present in malignant pathology. Retrosternal extension of a thyroid swelling may present with choking episodes and/or stridor.

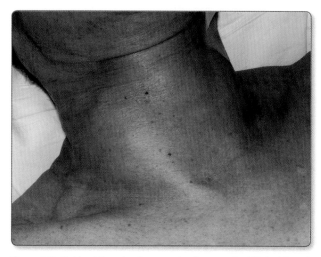

Figure 5.11 Multinodular goitre demonstrating the generalised bilobed thyroid gland swelling.

The different types of thyroid cancer and their prevalences are:
- Papillary and Mixed Papillary Follicular (Commonest) 78%
- Follicular and Hurthle Cell 17%
- Medullary 4%
- Anaplastic 1%.

Investigation

Thyroid function tests are usually done at primary care level. Most hypo- or hyperfunctioning goitres are benign.

The preferred investigation is ultrasound-guided fine-needle aspiration (FNA) cytology, the results of which are interpreted according to the British Thyroid Association guidelines into five groups as THY 1–5 (**Table 5.4**). Other investigations include technetium scanning (radioisotope uptake) and CT and MRI scans of the region, including the chest and mediastinum where appropriate.

If the FNA is suggestive of malignancy or is malignant, CT is the preferred investigation for evaluating retrosternal extension,

THY class	Description
THY1	Inadequate: repeat the ultrasound and FNA; if still non-diagnostic in the presence of solid tumour, then surgical excision indicated
THY2	Benign
THY3	Follicular lesion
THY4	Suspicious of malignancy
THY5	Malignant
FNA, fine-needle aspiration.	

Table 5.4 THY classification of thyroid FNA aspiration samples in suspected malignancy

cervical lymphadenopathy and the chest for staging and planning surgery. There is small chance of a false negative test (6%).

Diagnosis

The clinical features suggesting a referral is indicated ('red flags') include:

- A child with thyroid swelling
- Family history of thyroid cancer
- History of exposure to radiation
- Dysphonia and/or stridor with thyroid swelling
- Rapid increase in the size of the swelling over short period without any pain
- Associated neck lymphadenopathy.

Management

Guidelines for the management of thyroid cancer are outlined below.

Cancer units use the TNM (Tumour size, Nodal metastasis, distant Metastasis) classification for staging malignant disease and to analyse results between various centres. The most current staging system for each head and neck malignancy can be found in the document 'TNM Classification of Malignant tumours' available on the IUCC website (http://www.uicc.org/tnm).

Management is guided by the size of the swelling, the presence of associated symptoms, red flag symptoms and, more importantly, the THY grade. In a benign pathology, surgery is indicated for cosmetic purposes (a large goitre) and compression symptoms (e.g. choking episodes, coughing in the supine position). A thyroid nodule 1 cm or larger with suspicious features on ultrasound requires cytopathological evaluation to quantify the risk of malignancy.

Preoperative detection of malignancy ensures better counselling and management. Not all thyroid swellings need surgery. A benign goitre on ultrasound and FNA on two occasions at 6-month intervals can be discharged to primary care.

Medical

Hypo- or hyperfunctioning thyroid swellings are managed with thyroxine or anti-thyroid drugs under the supervision of the endocrinologist. Radioactive iodine is occasionally used to ablate overactive thyroid tissue under the supervision of a specialist in nuclear medicine.

Clinical insight

Molecular biomarkers are useful adjuvants to cytology:

- Papillary and medullary thyroid carcinoma are associated with mutations in the RAS, RET and BRAF genes
- Follicular thyroid cancer is associated with translocations between PAX 8 and PPAR-γ genes.

Surgical

Patients with a papillary carcinoma <1 cm can be adequately treated with lobectomy. Tumours >1 cm with multifocal disease require total thyroidectomy with neck clearance. For a follicular lesion THY3, lobectomy is mandatory for histopathological diagnosis. If the diagnosis is follicular carcinoma, complete thyroidectomy is indicated. Special mention must be made of medullary thyroid carcinoma because of the risk of other tumours both in the individual and in the family.

Prognosis

The risk of malignancy in a thyroid nodule is <4–7%. The prognosis for papillary and follicular carcinoma in younger patients, when treated early, is excellent. Medullary carcinoma has a tendency for early spread, and so requires aggressive treatment. Anaplastic carcinoma has the worst prognosis.

5.6 Salivary gland diseases

Salivary gland diseases include disorders of the major salivary glands (parotid, submandibular or sublingual) or minor salivary glands (600–1000 in number) dispersed throughout the upper aerodigestive submucosa (i.e. oral cavity, pharynx, larynx, parapharyngeal space, paranasal sinuses).

Epidemiology

Major salivary gland diseases are much more common than minor salivary gland disorders. The parotid glands (**Figure 5.12**) are affected more often than submandibular glands, and sublingual glands are the least affected.

Causes

A summary of the varied causes of salivary gland diseases is presented in **Table 5.5**.

Nearly 100% of sublingual, 80% of minor salivary gland, 50% of submandibular and 20% of parotid gland neoplasms are malignant.

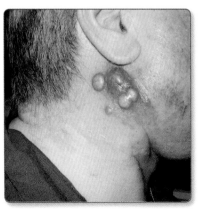

Figure 5.12 Malignant tumour of the right parotid gland with local spread to the overlying skin.

Infective	**Viral:** mumps, HIV, cytomegalovirus, Epstein-Barr virus, coxsackievirus, measles, echovirus **Acute bacterial:** *Staphylococcus aureus*, *Haemophilus influenzae*, *Streptococcus viridians* **Chronic bacterial:** acute infection as above, *Mycobacterium tuberculosis*, actinomycosis, *Bartonella henselae*, syphilis
Inflammatory	Sjögren's syndrome (salivary gland involvement is seen in 40% of cases, 33–44% of these develop lymphoma in later life) Sarcoidosis (parotid enlargement with facial nerve palsy and uveitis is Heerfordt's syndrome) Wegener's granulomatosis Juvenile recurrent parotitis (symptoms stop at puberty)
Neoplastic	**Benign:** pleomorphic adenoma (65% of all salivary tumours), papillary cystadenoma lymphomatosum (Warthin's tumour in 6–10% of all parotid tumours, with 10% bilateral) **Malignant (Figure 5.12):** mucoepidermoid carcinoma (commonest, 6–9% of all salivary gland cancers, parotid > submandibular), adenoid cystic carcinoma (second commonest, 6% of all salivary gland cancers, submandibular > parotid), carcinoma ex-pleomorphic adenoma (2–5% of all salivary gland tumours), acinic cell carcinoma, adenocarcinoma, metastasis
Degenerative	**Stone (sialolith):** submandibular gland/duct (80% of cases, 90% are radio-opaque), parotid (19% of cases, 90% are radiolucent), sublingual and minor salivary glands (1% of cases) **Cysts:** mucous extravasation cysts, mucous retention cysts and ranula (large mucous cyst of floor of mouth region) **Others:** amyloidosis, cirrhosis, Cushing's disease, diabetes, gout, bulimia, alcoholism, hypothyroidism and drugs, e.g. thiouracil

Table 5.5 Causes of salivary gland disease

Clinical features

A detailed history with a thorough review of systemic symptoms and drug history is essential. The commonest presenting symptom is swelling of the involved salivary glands. Other symptoms include:

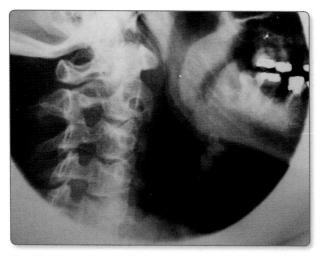

Figure 5.13 Submandibular gland with multiple calculi.

- mouth dryness
- halitosis
- pain or increased swelling with eating
- decreased mouth opening
- cranial nerve palsies (facial, lingual, hypoglossal)
- dryness of the eyes
- systemic symptoms in cases of infective and inflammatory pathology.

A thorough examination should include bimanual palpation of the salivary glands and their ducts, neck nodes, cranial nerve assessment, and nasendoscopy of the pharynx. Parotid swellings appear adjacent to the ear near the angle of the jaw; submandibular swellings appear below the mandible, and sublingual swellings in the floor of the mouth.

Acute infections usually result from ascending spread from the oral cavity or haematogenous spread. Dehydration or obstructed glands, malnutrition, immunosuppression and poor oral hygiene are predisposing factors. Painful swellings are usually infective or inflammatory in origin, although adenoid cystic carcinomas can cause pain. Painless swellings indicate a neoplastic, degenerative or chronic infective process.

Investigation

Haematological Haematological tests include FBC (showing raised WBC in infection), CRP (raised in presence of inflammation), ACE (raised in sarcoidosis), ANCA (positive c-ANCA, in Wegener's granulomatosis), serological tests for viruses including mumps and HIV, specific autoantibodies (Rho and La), and antinuclear antibodies and rheumatoid factor (suggesting Sjögren's syndrome).

Microbiology Pus is taken for microscopy, culture and guidance on antibiotic sensitivities.

Plain radiographs These are useful for calculus disease, especially of the submandibular glands (**Figure 5.13**).

Ultrasonography This is usually the first-line investigation, with FNA for investigation of a parotid/submandibular gland swelling.

CT/MRI Cross-sectional imaging is necessary for neoplastic disease to delineate the extent and spread of the tumour and plan resection.

Interventional sialography This can be used for direct evaluation of the ducts and also has the advantage of possible therapeutic intervention (balloon angiography, basket retrieval of calculi).

> ### Clinical insight
>
> Open biopsy is almost totally contraindicated in salivary gland swellings, the exception being neoplasms of the minor glands, as tumours spilt by biopsy will seed the area and result in the development of multiple recurrences within the biopsy scar. FNA biopsy is the method of choice.

Management

The specific management depends on the cause. Only a brief overview is presented here.

General measures include attention to oral hygiene (aided by an antiseptic mouthwash) and hydration to maintain good salivary flow.

- Acute viral infections require supportive treatment, although HIV requires specialist involvement
- Acute bacterial infection requires an broad-spectrum antibiotic covering aerobic and anaerobic organisms (e.g. co-amoxiclav); consider the intravenous route if there is systemic disturbance or difficulty taking oral fluids
- Abscesses may require incision and drainage, with careful regard to the facial nerve. Chronic infection such as TB should be referred to a chest physician for anti-tuberculous medication
- Inflammatory causes (e.g. Sjögren's, sarcoidosis, Wegener's) should be managed with the help of a rheumatologist as steroids and immune-modulating drugs will be required. Rarely parotidectomy or submandibular gland excision is needed for intractable swelling or pain associated with inflammatory diseases
- Salivary gland or duct stones may be retrieved with interventional sialography or require either local excision or gland excision together with the stone
- Patients with neoplastic lesions should be discussed in the multidisciplinary team meeting to agree an appropriate management plan.

> **Clinical insight**
>
> *Frey's syndrome* or gustatory sweating can occur after parotidectomy. There is redness and sweating on the ipsilateral face/neck when the patient smells, eats or even talks about food. This response is caused by regenerating parasympathetic fibres severed for salivary secretion inappropriately attaching to the sympathetic fibres in the skin

Prognosis

Benign salivary gland disease generally has a favourable outcome, although facial nerve compromise after parotidectomy can have considerable social and emotional impact. For malignant disease, the stage of disease at presentation (TNM classification) correlates the best with ultimate outcome.

5.7 Pharyngeal pouch

Pharyngeal pouches arise as a result of herniation of the posterior pharyngeal mucosa through a relatively unsupported part of the upper oesophageal sphincter. This weak part of the posterior pharyngeal wall, termed Killian's dehiscence, lies between the cricopharyngeus and thyropharyngeus.

Epidemiology

The outpouching of the pharyngeal mucosa is also referred to as posterior pharyngeal pulsion (Zenker's) diverticulum. The incidence is approximately 1 in 200 000 population per year. It occurs more commonly in elderly men than in women.

Causes and pathogenesis

The aetiology is unknown but the pathogenesis is probably multifactorial. Several theories, including weakness of the Killian's dehiscence, incoordination of the first (pharyngeal) phase of swallowing and an increase in intrapharyngeal pressure and cricopharyngeal muscle spasm, could be contributory factors. Hiatus hernia and gastro-oesophageal reflux are sometimes present.

As it enlarges the pouch becomes symptomatic; food can enter the pouch preferentially and in the later stages the pouch extends into the posterior mediastinum, exerting pressure on the oesophagus and resulting in dysphagia.

Clinical features

Small pouches may remain asymptomatic. The common presenting symptoms include a sensation of a lump in the throat, gradually worsening dysphagia and regurgitation of undigested food with halitosis. Weight loss and recurrent chest infection due to aspiration may prompt urgent referral. The swelling in the neck, usually on the left side, may gurgle and empty with external pressure.

Diseases restricting neck movements and limited jaw opening reduce surgical access and affect management. Elderly patients with recurrent chest infections and aspiration have a poor pulmonary reserve, adding to general anaesthetic risk.

Investigation

A plain **radiograph** of the neck and cervical spine may show an air-filled space in the pouch and the state of the cervical vertebrae. The definitive investigation is a **barium swallow (Figure 5.14)** that demonstrates the pouch. A rigid **oesophagoscopy** is carried out prior to surgical treatment to exclude carcinoma in the wall of the pouch.

Management

Asymptomatic patients may be treated with a conservative 'wait and watch' policy, as the pouch may remain static in size for quite some time. In symptomatic patients endoscopic stapling is the treatment of choice. However, difficult anatomy with limited neck extension, restricted jaw opening and protruding upper teeth may preclude endoscopic approaches. Small pouches are sometimes not amenable to endoscopic stapling if the amount of tissue separating the pouch from the pharynx (the 'bar') is too small for the staple gun to be engaged. Larger

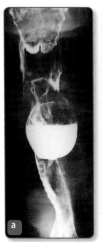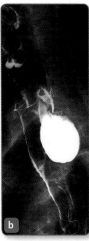

Figure 5.14 Barium swallow from the same sequence outlining a pharyngeal pouch. In (a) the barium has half-filled the pouch and in (b) the pouch is fully filled.

pouches are clearly visualised (**Figure 5.15**) and a thorough inspection to exclude carcinoma is carried out before stapling and dividing the bar between the pouch and the oesophagus (**Figure 5.16**).

The main disadvantage of endoscopic surgery is that the pouch is not excised but opened into the oesophagus to allow the passage of food. The advantages of endoscopic stapling, however, far outweigh the risks:

- Reduced surgical time and hospital stay
- Avoids suture lines in the neck and oesophagus
- Significantly reduces the risk compared to open procedures.

In patients in whom endoscopic techniques have failed or have not been possible because of anatomical factors, open procedures are used. This could be a diverticulotomy, where the pouch is excised, combined with myotomy of the crico-pharyngeal muscles. Some surgeons do not excise the sac but

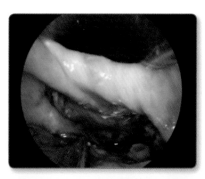

Figure 5.15 Endoscopic view of the bar between the pharyngeal pouch (seen posteriorly) and the oesophagus (anteriorly).

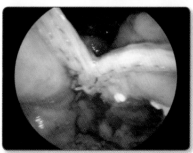

Figure 5.16 Endoscopic view following stapling of the bar: the pouch wall is incorporated as part of the wider oesophageal wall.

invert and oversew the pouch to avoid the risk of opening and suturing the oesophagus. Nasogastric feeding is required for 5–7 days postoperatively.

Prognosis

The majority of patients improve symptomatically following endoscopic stapling; a small proportion (<8–10%) who remain symptomatic may require a second stapling procedure. Quality of life improves following surgical treatment, with the ability to eat all types of food and the prevention of aspiration and recurrent chest infections.

5.8 Benign neck lumps

Neck lumps may be solitary or multiple. They may be classified as congenital or acquired, benign or malignant. Only benign neck lumps are considered in this chapter.

Causes

Causes of benign neck lumps are shown in **Table 5.6**.

Clinical features

Neck lumps may present as asymptomatic swellings first noticed while shaving (in men) or looking in the mirror, or they

Congenital	
Midline	Lateral
Thyroglossal duct cyst	Branchial cyst
Dermoid cyst	Haemangioma
	Lymphangiomatous malformation
Acquired	
Inflammatory	Neoplastic
Infective: bacterial, viral, fungal, parasitic, deep neck space infection	Lipoma, neurofibroma
Non-infective: Sarcoidosis, Wegener's granulomatosis	Paraganglioma
	Salivary/thyroid gland tumours

Table 5.6 Causes of a benign neck lump

present with pain, tenderness or rapid growth. Important features from the history include:

- smoking
- weight loss
- fever or night sweats
- recent upper respiratory infection
- drug use
- recent contact history or travel abroad
- associated symptoms of ear pain, sore throat, dysphagia, dysphonia or breathing difficulty.

Clinical examination of the anterior and posterior triangles of the neck should include all lymph node levels as well as the thyroid and major salivary glands. Examination of the ears, nose and throat should include a fibreoptic nasendoscopy and examination of the skin of the scalp to avoid missing a possible primary site.

> ## Clinical insight
>
> *Ludwig's angina* is a deep neck space infection of the sublingual and submandibular spaces, usually arising from a dental source. The patient presents with tender swelling of the floor of mouth and upper midline neck which can compromise the airway. Treatment is to secure the airway and administer antibiotics.

Investigations

The primary investigation of a neck lump is an ultrasound scan with **FNA** biopsy. The scan will help localise the site of pathology as well as determine whether the swelling is solid or cystic. Expert radiologists can also comment with a high level of confidence whether a lymph node is reactive or warrants biopsy or further imaging. CT with contrast is especially useful to investigate a neck abscess or deep neck space infection. MRI gives superior soft tissue detail and is useful for imaging congenital, vascular or neoplastic swellings.

Blood tests are indicated when an infective or inflammatory lymphadenitis is suspected. As well as FBC and CRP, specific tests include ACE (sarcoidosis), c-ANCA (Wegener's granulomatosis), Quantiferon-TB Gold (tuberculosis), anti-SSA and anti-SSB (Sjögren's syndrome) and serological antibody tests (EBV, HIV, toxoplasmosis, cat scratch disease, mumps).

Management

For a reactive neck gland all that may be required is reassurance and monitoring. Treatment for a specific infective cause is tailored to the specific pathogen and will not be formally discussed here. Neck lymphadenitis caused by sarcoidosis or Wegener's granulomatosis should be discussed with the rheumatologist, as some form of immune-modulating drugs are needed, requiring their experience. Thyroid lumps (p. 175), salivary gland lumps (p. 179) and thyroglossal cysts (p. 218) are discussed elsewhere. Some useful considerations for managing specific neck lumps are considered below.

> **Clinical insight**
>
> A lateral cystic neck mass presenting after the age of 40 in a smoker should not be presumed to be a branchial cyst. Careful examination and investigation should evaluate the possibility of a primary malignancy in the head and neck region before excision is considered.

Dermoid cysts

These originate from ectoderm and mesoderm and the majority present by 5 years of age. They occur in the midline but do not move on swallowing or tongue protrusion, and contain skin appendages such as hair follicles, sebaceous glands and sweat glands. Treatment is complete surgical excision.

Branchial/lateral cervical cysts

Clinical presentation is discussed on p. 156. They are thought to arise from elements of squamous epithelium within a lymph node, although other suggestions include remnants of the first pharyngeal pouch, a cervical sinus, or the duct connecting the thymus to the third pharyngeal pouch. They commonly present in late childhood or early adulthood, usually after an upper respiratory tract infection. They are predominantly left-sided and lie anterior to the upper border of sternocleidomastoid. FNA helps in diagnosis and shows a straw-coloured fluid. Aspiration and antibiotics may be required if there is acute infection, although definitive management is complete surgical excision (**Figure 5.17**).

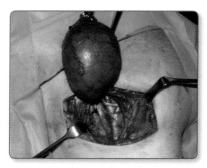

Figure 5.17 Right branchial cyst.

Lymphangiomatous malformations

These are congenital malformations of the lymphatic system, which can be broadly divided into microcystic and macrocystic types, although the traditional terms of capillary, cavernous and cystic hygroma are still used. Microcystic lesions usually arise in the lips, cheek and floor of the mouth, whereas macrocystic lesions usually arise in the lower neck. Surgical excision is the mainstay of treatment, although sclerosants (OK-432 and hypertonic saline), cryotherapy, cautery and CO_2 laser vaporisation have been used. Propranolol represents a potential new option, which may be of benefit even for intractable diffuse lymphangiomatosis.

Paragangliomas

Paragangliomas are neoplasms that arise from extra-adrenal paraganglia. Carotid body and glomus tumours can present as painless pulsatile neck masses in the upper deep cervical region, sometimes with lower cranial nerve palsies in tumours extending up to the skull base; 10–20% present with multiple paragangliomas and 5% are malignant. Magnetic resonance angiography (MRA) aids diagnosis. Treatment is surgical excision, although radiotherapy may be offered to arrest growth in the elderly or where there are significant risks of functional compromise.

5.9 Cancer of the oral cavity and pharynx

Cancer of the oral cavity and the pharynx arises mainly from the mucosal lining of the respective anatomical region. Oral cancers include those arising from the cheek, oral tongue (anterior two thirds), floor of mouth, hard palate, alveolar ridges and lip. The term pharyngeal cancer includes cancers arising in various pharyngeal sub-sites such as the oropharynx, nasopharynx and hypopharynx. The behaviour and prognosis of the lesions differ according to the sub-site involved.

Epidemiology

The incidence of oral and pharyngeal cancers varies immensely (0.5 – 41 per 100 000 population) depending on the geographical region, age and gender of the patient, and sub-site of origin of the disease. The incidence rates of oral cavity and pharyngeal cancers among males in the UK are 10.0 and 2.5 per 100 000 population, respectively. The disease is more commonly seen in males (M:F = 2:1 to 5:1) and is more common in the sixth and seventh decades. However, recent trends suggest a shift in age towards the younger population and a sharp rise in women because of increasing smoking trends.

Causes and pathogenesis

The aetiology of oral and pharyngeal cancers is multifactorial. Lifestyle factors that contribute to a higher incidence include:

- tobacco smoking
- alcohol
- betel quid and areca nut chewing
- oral sex (HPV transmission).

Other risk factors are:

- viruses (HPV, EBV, HIV)
- genetic factors
- dietary deficiencies (especially of fruits and antioxidants)
- environmental factors and occupational exposure
- immunosuppression

- chronic irritation of the mucosa either by exposure to carcinogens or by repeated trauma (e.g. a sharp tooth).

It is a preventable disease and 80% of cases can be avoided by simply modifying lifestyle habits.

Clinical features

The clinical presentation depends on the site of the cancer (**Table 5.7**). The common presentations of oral cancer include:

- Painless swelling
- Proliferative growth
- Irregular area of cracking or fissuring
- Localised discoloration (reddish or whitish)
- Frank non-healing ulcer of recent onset (**Figure 5.18**).

Pain is a late symptom and indicates an advanced stage of disease. Other common presentations are excessive salivation, occasional bleeding/streaking from the mouth, loosening of teeth and difficulty in chewing, altered speech or a recent-onset swelling in the neck (metastasis).

Type of cancer	Presentation
Oropharyngeal	Neck swelling (metastasis) Foreign body sensation/soreness Discomfort in the throat, especially on swallowing Otalgia Altered speech (lump in the throat) Halitosis Decreased tongue mobility affecting speech and swallowing
Nasopharyngeal	Although a pharyngeal subsite, this tumour has been discussed in the section on sinonasal tumours (p. 148)
Hypopharyngeal	Neck swelling Unilateral foreign body sensation/soreness/ discomfort Food sticking in the throat, especially on swallowing Recent change in voice (due to laryngeal involvement) Unintentional weight loss

Table 5.7 Clinical presentation of different types of oral cancers

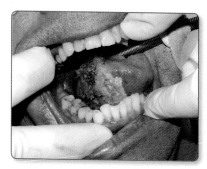

Figure 5.18 Squamous cell carcinoma of the right lateral border of the tongue.

A high index of suspicion is required: high-risk patients (smokers, tobacco users, alcoholics) presenting with symptoms of recent onset (weeks/months) with or without recent weight loss must be referred urgently to a head and neck surgeon.

Investigation and diagnosis

Meticulous ENT examination is essential. The first step is to confirm the diagnosis, which is established by histopathological examination of the suspected lesion. Tissue is generally taken by performing biopsy under local anaesthesia if the lesion is superficial and approachable and the patient is cooperative, or under general anaesthesia in all other situations. In cases presenting with only neck metastasis ultrasound-guided FNA cytology should be done first to ascertain the malignant nature of the disease, subsequently proceeding to locate the primary lesion and obtain a tissue diagnosis.

The next step is to ascertain the spread (local and/or distant) of the disease and to stage the cancer, as the management and prognosis depend on the stage of the disease. Staging investigations include panendoscopy and examination under general anaesthesia, CT and/or MRI scans of the head, neck and chest, and in some cases positron emission tomography (PET)/bone scans may be required. The most current staging system for each head and neck malignancy can be found in the document 'TNM Classification of Malignant tumours' available

> ## Clinical insight
>
> The multidisciplinary team includes a head and neck surgeon, radiologist, pathologist, radiation oncologist, medical oncologist, plastic and reconstructive surgeons, dental oncologist/prosthodontist, speech and swallowing therapist, clinical nurse specialist, dietician and clinical social worker.

on the IUCC website (http://www.uicc.org/tnm).

As well as diagnostic and staging examination/investigations, detailed nutritional assessment, medical evaluation and psychosocial assessment help in deciding optimal management for the individual patient. This is a complex, multistage process and involves many experts from diverse specialties working together in a multidisciplinary team.

Management

These cancers can be managed by surgery, radiotherapy, chemotherapy or any combination of these, depending on the stage of disease. A multidisciplinary team approach is essential.

Early-stage (stages I and II) cancers can be effectively managed by a single treatment modality (surgery or radiotherapy) with nearly equal results, whereas advanced-stage (stage III or IV) disease usually requires combined modalities. Surgery is generally preferred over radiotherapy for oral cancers (irrespective of the stage of disease), and radiotherapy is preferred for nasopharyngeal and hypopharyngeal cancers irrespective of stage as well as late-stage oropharyngeal cancers. For early-stage oropharyngeal cancers surgery and radiotherapy are equally effective.

Prognosis

The prognosis depends on the site and stage of the disease at the time of initial presentation and the chosen treatment modality. Early presentation has a better prognosis than late, and oral cavity cancers have better prognoses than the pharyngeal cancers. Most patients require long-term follow-up and functional rehabilitation in order to achieve a good quality of life after treatment.

5.10 Cancer of the larynx

Cancer of the larynx commonly arises from its mucosal lining, and therefore is predominantly of squamous cell type (90%). Based on the anatomical sub-site of origin, it can be divided into glottic (69%), supraglottic (27%) or subglottic (4%). Each region has its own peculiar presentation and outcomes.

Epidemiology

The global incidence varies between 2.5 and 17.2 per 100 000 population. For males and females in the UK these rates are 5.3 and 1.0 per 100 000 population, respectively. Three-quarters of cases are seen in people over 60 years of age. In the younger population the incidence rates in males and females are nearly equal.

Causes and pathogenesis

The aetiology is multifactorial, with lifestyle playing the most crucial role. It is a preventable disease. The commonest risk factors include tobacco smoking and/or alcohol. Environmental, genetic and dietary factors, socioeconomic status and occupational exposure to carcinogens also play a role.

Clinical features

The commonest presenting symptom is hoarseness, which occurs early in cases of glottic cancers but not in supra- or subglottic cancers. Other important symptoms are:

- dyspnoea
- noisy breathing
- stridor (early in subglottic and glottic, late in supraglottic cancers),
- chronic cough
- blood-streaked sputum
- haemoptysis from bleeding, ulcerative or proliferative lesions (**Figure 5.19**)
- sore throat

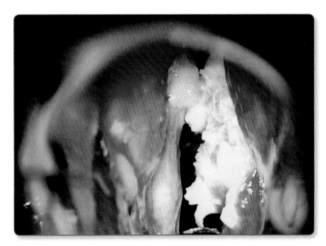

Figure 5.19 Proliferative lesion of the right vocal fold.

- odynophagia/dysphagia
- neck lump (from secondary spread to a cervical lymph node, especially for supraglottic cancers).

A detailed history and thorough ENT examination (including flexible nasoendoscopy (FNE) and neck examination) are essential. A high index of suspicion is needed, especially with high-risk patients (smokers, tobacco users, alcoholics). Symptoms of short duration/recent onset must be taken seriously, and patients should be urgently referred to ENT for a specialist opinion and work-up.

Investigation

As with any other head and neck cancer the definitive diagnosis is established by histopathological examination of the suspected lesion. Microlaryngoscopy and biopsy is performed and, if possible, panendoscopy and examination under anaesthesia at the same time. This helps in correctly staging the disease and can detect any second primary tumours. To evaluate the extent of the disease (staging) US of the neck with or without FNAC, CT/MRI of the head, neck and chest, and in advanced-stage lesions (if deemed necessary) PET/bone scans may be needed. Each head and neck malignancy can be found in the document 'TNM Classification of Malignant tumours' available on the IUCC website (http://www.uicc.org/tnm).

Management

Laryngeal cancers can be managed by any of the approaches outlined below, depending on patient factors (age, general health and co-morbidities, occupation, personal/social and lifestyle considerations) disease factors (histological type, grade and extent/stage of disease) and clinician factors (availability of resources and personal preferences).

Management options include:

- Conservative laryngeal surgery in the form of endoscopic transoral laser surgery
- Open partial laryngectomy
- Total laryngectomy
- Radiotherapy alone or combined with chemoradiation.

Conservative approaches are preferred for early-stage (stage I and II) lesions, whereas more radical approaches are adopted for advanced-stage (stage III and IV) cancers. As a rule all decisions regarding patient management are made by a multidisciplinary team.

Loss of normal laryngeal function is the most important complication and may have a crippling effect on patients' psychosocial function. Therefore, treatment should be individualised for every patient, depending on the factors mentioned above. Patients should be followed up and rehabilitated by the team, especially with speech and swallowing therapists. They should also be encouraged to participate in focused group activities.

Prognosis

The outcome depends on the sub-site(s) involved, disease stage and the type of treatment used. In general, glottic cancers have the best prognosis and supraglottic cancers the worst, irrespective of the treatment modality used. Overall 5-year survival rates for early and late stage cancers range from 80–95% and 40–60%, respectively.

5.11 Snoring and obstructive sleep apnoea

Obstructive sleep-disordered breathing is a spectrum of diseases ranging from simple snoring to obstructive sleep apnoea syndrome (OSAS): Simple snoring →Upper airway resistance syndrome (UARS) → Mild OSAS→ Moderate OSAS→ Severe OSAS. The definitions of these diseases are:

- **Snoring:** noisy breathing due to partial obstruction and vibration of the respiratory structures in the oral cavity and/or pharynx (e.g. soft palate)
- **Upper airway resistance syndrome (UARS):** snoring in the presence of airway resistance to breathing, which is associated with daytime somnolence and excessive fatigue. Unlike OSA, women are as likely as men to have UARS and sufferers tend to have normal weight
- **Obstructive sleep apnoea (OSA):** a serious, potentially life-threatening condition associated with repetitive episodes of complete (apnoea) or partial (hypopnoea) obstruction of the upper airway during sleep
- **Obstructive sleep apnoea syndrome (OSAS):** OSA in combination with symptoms such as daytime somnolence and excessive fatigue. It has potential consequences for patients and their partners (**Table 5.8**). Its aetiology is multifactorial, with various risk factors (**Table 5.9**).

Epidemiology

The prevalence of habitual snoring is 30–50% and for OSAS is 2–4%. The male:female ratio is 2:1. Approximately 50% of patients with OSAS are obese (body mass index ≥ 30 kg/m^2).

Clinical features

History and examination should aim to identify and assess the severity of obstructive sleep disorder, risk factors for OSAS (see **Table 5.9**) and any secondary consequences (which can vary from psychosocial problems to cardiovascular consequences). History should include:

Patient	
Social	**Impaired social functioning**
Neurocognitive	Unrefreshing sleep Excessive daytime somnolence Excessive tiredness Headache Reduced libido Poor concentration Personality change/irritability Accident at work Road traffic accident
Multisystem	30% of patients with hypertension have OSAS 30% of patients with OSAS have hypertension 10% develop cor pulmonale May increase risk of stroke and myocardial infarction
Partner	
	Poor sleep hygiene Reduced libido Marital problems Stress

Table 5.8 Potential consequences of obstructive sleep apnoea (OSAS)

- Male gender
- Increasing age
- Obesity (BMI $\geq$ 30 kg/m^2)
- Neck circumference 17 inches
- Hypertension
- Alcohol/sedative drugs
- Craniofacial abnormality
- Positive family history

Table 5.9 Risk factors for obstructive sleep apnoea

- sleeping pattern
- observed apnoeic episodes
- choking events
- reflux
- drugs (in particular sleeping tablets and antidepressants)
- alcohol intake

- smoking
- job/shift pattern
- past medical history, including depression, sexual dysfunction, hypothyroidism, cardiopulmonary diseases, diabetes, acromegaly, Down's syndrome and Marfan's syndrome.

In the examination, associated signs include:

- tonsil and adenoid hypertrophy
- macroglossia
- micro- or retrognathia
- redundant pharyngeal mucosa
- crowded oropharynx
- craniofacial abnormalities
- large neck size
- nasal, pharyngeal or laryngeal obstruction.

Investigation

Epworth sleepiness scale (ESS)

Although correlation between the Epworth sleepiness scale (ESS) and severity of OSAS is relatively weak, ESS is the best-validated questionnaire and reflects patients' perception of their sleepiness. The maximum score is 24 and ESS < 11 is considered normal.

Polysomnography

Polysomnography (PSG) is the gold standard test for diagnosing sleep apnoea. All patients with symptoms or signs suggestive of OSA and/or a subjective measure of daytime somnolence (ESS >10) should at least have a limited sleep study.

The apnoea–hypopnoea index (AHI)

This is an index of the severity of OSAS based on the number of apnoea plus hypopnoea episodes per hour of sleep (AHI 5–20 mild OSA, 21–41 moderate OSA, >40 severe OSA).

Sleep nasendoscopy

Sleep nasendoscopy is used in some units. Although this is drug-induced sleep, it may give some useful information about the level of obstruction and help plan treatment.

Additional investigations

Depending on the clinical findings, investigations such as thyroid function (for hypothyroidism), full blood count (for polycythemia), chest radiography (for cor pulmonale) and flow–volume loops (for airways disease) are requested.

Management

Treatment for simple snoring varies from reassurance, advice about sleep hygiene and sleeping position to weight loss, a mandibular advancement splint (MAS), palatal radiofrequency, palatal implant and uvulo-palatoplasty.

The commonest form of palatal surgery is laser-assisted uvulo-palatoplasty (LAUP), which aims to shorten and stiffen the soft palate (**Figure 5.20**). Sometimes partners can resolve the

> ### Clinical insight
>
> Patients with OSAS need ongoing help and support to deal with any issues with nasal CPAP, otherwise compliance will be poor. A frequent problem can be 'CPAP rhinitis', which can usually be managed with a topical steroid nasal spray.
>
> Adults with OSAS who require tonsillectomy should be advised to bring in their CPAP machine to help in the postoperative period. They should be kept in hospital overnight and there should be provision for admission to a high-dependency unit if needed postoperatively

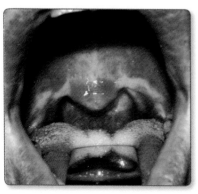

Figure 5.20 Postoperative appearance following LAUP surgery, demonstrating a shortened and stiffened palate (neo-uvula).

Behavioural advice	Weight loss and exercise Alcohol avoidance Avoidance of sedative medications
Non-surgical	CPAP (gold standard) Mandibular advancement splint for mild OSAS
Surgical	Nasal surgery (facilitate use of nasal CPAP) Tonsillectomy (if large tonsils) Tracheostomy Mandibular and maxillary advancement Genioglossal advancement and hyoid suspension Bariatric surgery (provoke weight loss)
CPAP: continuous positive airway pressure	

Table 5.10 Management options for obstructive sleep apnoea syndrome (OSAS)

problem by wearing ear plugs or having the radio on at night.

OSAS requires a multidisciplinary team approach which may include respiratory medicine, ENT surgery, maxillofacial surgery, orthodontics and dietetics. Treatments include behavioural, non-surgical and surgical options (**Table 5.10**). The gold standard therapy for moderate/severe OSAS is nasal continuous positive airway pressure (CPAP).

In patients with OSAS the ability to drive can be affected. Therefore, they should be advised to inform the DVLA and avoid driving until a specialist confirms that their condition is controlled.

Prognosis
Simple snoring, although not life-threatening, can have serious consequences, such as marital break-up. Untreated OSAS can have potential serious cardiovascular consequences, but adequately treated OSAS has a good prognosis.

6.1 Clinical scenarios

Rhinorrhoea

Background

A 4-year-old boy had presented with a previous history of upper respiratory tract infection, featuring an itchy, runny nose and cough. His general practitioner had initially treated these with antibiotics and antihistamines and there was some improvement in the symptoms, but the discharge from the right nostril continued. The rhinorrhoea was initially mucoid and after 1 week became thick, greenish and foul-smelling, and was also occasionally bloodstained. The parents noticed that their son was constantly rubbing his nose and had been increasingly irritable over the last few days. They denied witnessing their child inserting any objects into his nose.

The GP prescribed some saline nose drops for the rhinorrhoea and subsequently added flucloxacillin. Two weeks after the initial visit to the GP, the discharge from the right nostril was still offensive-smelling and purulent, so the parents took him to the emergency department.

> **Clinical insight**
>
> An otoscope is useful to examine the nose of a young child.

History

The boy was born prematurely and has autism and eczema. Both his parents suffer with allergic rhinitis.

Examination

The child was extremely anxious and reluctant to be examined, although there were no signs of respiratory distress. He was wrapped in a blanket to gently restrain his arms, and seated on his father's lap with the paediatric nurse helping to steady his head for nasal examination. The entrance of the

Clinical insight

Unilateral nasal discharge in a child is caused by a foreign body until proven otherwise.

right nostril was found to be inflamed and there was a shiny metallic object with mucopus filling the right nasal cavity (**Figure 6.1**). On the left side there was a mild degree of rhinitis but no mucopus or vestibulitis.

Investigation

A microbiology swab of the nasal discharge was sent by the GP and cultured *Staphylococcus aureus*, which was sensitive to flucloxacillin.

Differential diagnosis

- **Foreign body**: unilateral nasal symptoms in a small child should place this high on the differential diagnosis list
- **Rhinosinusitis**: this is usually associated with purulent nasal discharge and obstruction
- **Allergic rhinitis**: this is common in children (1 in 4) with nasal block, itch, sneezing and rhinorrhoea
- **Structural anomalies**, such as deviated nasal septum, choanal atresia and adenoid hypertrophy can present with unilateral nasal symptoms in children
- **Tumour**: benign and malignant neoplasm of the nasal cavity is a possibility, though is very rare in children.

Discussion

The diagnosis here is a foreign body in the nose. There may also be a background of allergic rhinitis, which is common in

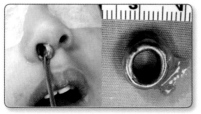

Figure 6.1 Foreign body in right nostril.

children, although this will not give unilateral symptoms. After gently restraining the child in a blanket, there should be one attempt at removal. Further attempts should be avoided, as this will only traumatise the child and be difficult. A short general anaesthetic may be required to facilitate removal.

Clinical insight

A button battery in the nose of a child must be removed urgently as leakage of alkaline fluid can cause considerable tissue necrosis and local damage.

Discharging ear
Background

A 4-year-old boy developed an upper respiratory tract infection with symptoms of runny nose, sore throat and mild fever. He was treated by his parents with paracetamol. After 2 days he developed purulent rhinorrhoea and complained of left-sided earache. His parents took him to the GP, who diagnosed left acute otitis media and prescribed a course of amoxicillin (125 mg three times daily for 5 days). He took the antibiotic for the first 3 days and then stopped because he developed diarrhoea. Initially, the rhinorrhoea and earache improved, but after a few days the boy developed a high temperature with increasing left earache, followed by yellowish ear discharge. The parents noticed that he was rather irritable and that his left ear was protruding forward. He was referred to the local ENT department as an emergency.

History

The boy is generally healthy but has not had the Hib vaccine owing to parental anxiety after reading an article on a possible link with juvenile diabetes. He has had recurrent viral upper respiratory tract infections (URTIs) since starting nursery school. His parents smoke at home.

Examination

On reaching the hospital the boy is pyrexial, with a temperature of 40 °C. The parents comment that he is not his usual playful self and is reluctant to eat. There is mucopus filling the left ear canal and a fluctuant tender swelling in the left postauricular region which has obliterated the postauricular sulcus (**Figure 6.2**). The skin overlying this swelling is erythematous. Examination of the nose shows generally rhinitic nasal mucosa.

Investigation

Blood tests show raised white blood cell count (WBC) of 28 x 10^9 cells/L, with predominant neutrophilia and raised C-reactive protein (CRP) of 180 mg/L. A microbiology swab taken from the ear discharge subsequently cultures *Haemophilus influenzae*. A CT scan of the temporal bones with intravenous contrast is urgently arranged after discussion with the duty radiologist, and shows opacification of the left middle ear cleft with disruption of the mastoid cortex and a surrounding non-enhancing soft tissue swelling. There is no associated intracranial abnormality.

Differential diagnosis

- **Otitis externa** with reactive postauricular lymphadenopathy
- **Acute otitis media with suppurative postauricular lymph node**

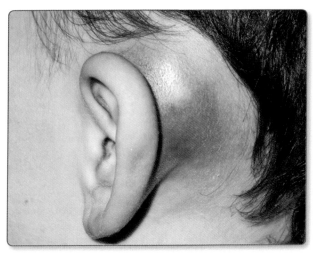

Figure 6.2 Acute otitis media with mastoiditis.

- **Acute otitis media with complicated mastoiditis**
- **Chronic otitis media** (cholesteatoma) with complicated mastoiditis
- **Acute mastoiditis** with associated intracranial complication, e.g. extradural abscess, subdural abscess, intracerebral abscess, meningitis
- *Rarely* Wegener's granulomatosis, leukaemia or histiocytosis.

> ## Clinical insight
>
> Intracranial complications are not uncommon with acute mastoiditis, so a high level of suspicion is needed. CT and MRI provide fast, accurate diagnosis of intracranial complications, but help from the paediatric team may be needed for lumbar puncture if meningitis is suspected.

Discussion

The diagnosis is acute otitis media with complicated mastoiditis. An upper respiratory infection will not just cause inflammation of the mucous membranes of the nose, but can also affect the mucous membranes of the paranasal sinuses and middle ear cleft. Where there may have been inadequate antibiotic dose or duration of treatment, antibiotic-resistant bacteria or an immunocompromised state, the risk of complications increases. Unfortunately, in this case, because of diarrhoea the antibiotic was stopped early and the infection spread, causing a mastoid abscess. Treatment is incision and drainage of the mastoid abscess, with myringotomy and grommet insertion under general anaesthesia.

Sore throat
Description

For the fifth time in 12 months a 6-year-old girl developed a sore throat. This was associated with pyrexia (38.1°C) and odynophagia. She felt too unwell to attend school. She was treated by her parents with paracetamol. After

> ## Clinical insight
>
> Antibiotics in otitis media:
>
> - Watchful waiting is reasonable in uncomplicated cases; however, if the child fails to improve within 2–3 days or there is a severe infection, antibiotics should be started
> - Indicators to prompt earlier prescription include high fever, vomiting, severe otalgia and age under 2 years
> - Local antibiotic policy should be followed, taking into account local antibiotic resistance.

2 days they took her to see their GP who diagnosed bacterial tonsillitis and prescribed penicillin V (250 mg four times daily), which the girl took for 3 days but without improvement. She developed some bilateral tender neck swelling and a left-sided earache. Because of the sore throat she was finding it difficult to swallow. She was refusing her medications and was gradually becoming dehydrated due to poor oral intake. Three days into the 7-day course of penicillin V she was referred to the local ENT department as an emergency.

History

Apart from her recurrent sore throats the girl is generally well. She snores every night and frequently has a blocked nose with mouth breathing. She previously suffered from apnoeas during her sleep but these have reduced with time, and her mother states that they only now occur when she has a URTI.

Her elder sister has had a tonsillectomy for recurrent tonsillitis. Her father is a smoker. He smokes in their flat, which also accommodates her mother and several other children. There is damp in the walls. Her sister suffers from multiple allergies and has recurrent lower respiratory tract infections. The school has become concerned about her multiple episodes of non-attendance.

Examination

On reaching hospital the girl is pyrexial, with a temperature of 38.2 °C. She appears tired and dehydrated and speaks infrequently, as she finds it uncomfortable. Her voice is slightly muffled. She has not passed urine in the last 7 hours. She finds swallowing her saliva painful but is not drooling.

Examination of the oropharynx demonstrates enlarged grade IV tonsils covered in white exudates (**Figure 6.3**). The uvula is central. She has mild trismus and prefers not to open her mouth widely. She has enlarged jugulodigastric nodes bilaterally which are tender. There is no hepatosplenomegaly. Despite her otalgia, ear examination is normal.

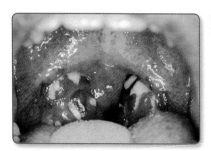

Figure 6.3 Acute tonsillitis.

Investigation

Blood tests show a raised WBC of 17×10^9/L with a predominant neutrophilia and a raised CRP of 119 mg/L. There are no abnormal leukocytes. A glandular fever test is negative. Urea and electrolytes and liver function tests are within normal limits.

Differential diagnosis

- **Viral tonsillitis**: this tends to be more self-limiting with milder symptoms, and is usually managed by analgesia and good fluid intake
- **Bacterial tonsillitis**: there is more systemic upset and inability to continue usual activities. Antibiotics are usually required
- **Bacterial tonsillitis with peritonsillar cellulitis or abscess**: a quinsy is very painful and gives rise to a 'hot potato' voice with some degree of associated trismus. The uvula will be pushed to the opposite side by the peritonsillar swelling
- **Bacterial tonsillitis with parapharyngeal cellulitis or abscess**: very rarely tonsil infection can spread locally to the parapharyngeal space

Clinical insight

The history can help differentiate the cause of a sore throat:

- *Tonsillitis* usually has associated fever, significant odynophagia, general malaise and disruption of normal activities
- *Pharyngitis* generally does not cause much systemic upset, or affect swallowing or normal activities.

- **Bacterial tonsillitis with retropharyngeal cellulitis or abscess**: very rarely tonsil infection can spread locally to the retropharyngeal space.

Discussion

The diagnosis here is acute bacterial tonsillitis. Management should be admission to hospital for intravenous fluids and antibiotics as well as adequate analgesia. The antibiotic of choice is benzylpenicillin, as the most likely pathogen is a group A *Streptococcus*. As there have been five episodes in the past year, with a significant episode requiring admission, an interval tonsillectomy after 6 weeks should be advised.

6.2 Otitis media with effusion

Otitis media with effusion is the chronic accumulation of mucus within the middle ear cleft (**Figure 6.4**). Chronic is usually defined when this has been present for more than 12 weeks.

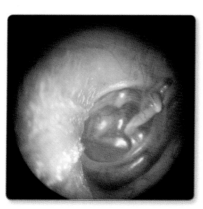

Figure 6.4 Otitis media with effusion and severe retraction of the tympanic membrane.

Epidemiology

Up to 40% of infants have had an episode of otitis media with effusion, reducing to 15% of 5-year-olds and 1% of 11-year-olds. There is therefore a natural tendency to resolution with increasing age. It is twice as likely to occur in the winter months as in the summer months.

Causes

Primarily there is dysfunction of the Eustachian tube. Several factors may contribute:
- Passive smoking, with oedema and impairment of ciliary function
- Chronic sinonasal or nasopharyngeal infection
- Adenoidal hypertrophy
- Craniofacial abnormalities, e.g. Down's or Turner's syndromes
- Disorder of the palatine muscles, e.g. cleft palate
- Gastro-oesophageal reflux.

Pathogenesis

Ventilation of the middle ear occurs via the Eustachian tube, which is lined by ciliated pseudostratified columnar epithelium. These cells, together with goblet cells and mucus-secreting glands, can result in the accumulation of middle ear mucus. A combination of oedema and inflammation of this lining and impaired Eustachian tube function, with negative middle ear pressure, can lead to failure of this fluid to drain.

Clinical features

The clinical features are listed in **Table 6.1**.

Investigation

Typical investigation findings in otitis media are summarised in **Table 6.2**.

Diagnosis

The diagnosis of otitis media with effusion is based on an appropriate history in conjunction with appropriate otoscopy, tympanometry and audiometry findings.

Clinical feature	Presentation
Hearing loss	May have been noticed with the TV volume turned up loud, child raising their voice, or through concerns reported from school
Speech and language delay	Good hearing is necessary for normal development of speech and language
Behavioural problems	
Inattentive or hyperactive child	
Recurrent earaches with repeated ear infections	
Adenoidal hypertrophy	Snoring, nasal obstruction and mouth breathing
Clumsiness	Can occur in up to 30% of children, although the exact mechanism is uncertain
Tinnitus	Rarely reported

Table 6.1 Clinical features of otitis media with effusion

Diagnostic test	Results
Otoscopy	Appearances are variable; features include colour changes, congestion, retraction and fluid levels of the tympanic membrane (**Figure 6.4**)
Tympanometry	Interpret findings in conjunction with otoscopy and audiometry. With increasing likelihood of an effusion the following may be seen: • Peak between –100 and –199 daPa (type C1) • Peak between –200 and –399 (type C2) • Flat trace (type b)
Audiogram	An age-appropriate hearing test should be performed in all suspected cases

Table 6.2 Results of investigations in otitis media with effusion

Management

There is NICE guidance on the management of otitis media with effusion (see **Appendix**).

Prognosis

In around 50% of children who are referred into secondary care with bilateral otitis media with effusion, the problem resolves with a watchful waiting period of 3 months. Of those with persistent effusions that require grommet insertion (**Figure 6.5**) up to 25% may require a second set of grommets.

There is a potential risk that chronic otitis media with effusion and persisting poor Eustachian tube function could lead to attic retractions and the development of cholesteatoma, although the true incidence of this is not known. Tympanosclerosis and atrophy of the tympanic membrane can also occur with otitis media with effusion, or be a sequela of grommet insertion (**Figure 6.6**). Long-term significant hearing problems are unusual in adequately treated or resolved otitis media with effusion.

6.3 Adenotonsillar disease

Adenotonsillar disease in children is mainly attributable to infection or hypertrophy of the adenoids and tonsils **(Figure 6.7)**, which can give rise to partial airway obstruction (obstructive sleep apnoea or blocked nose).

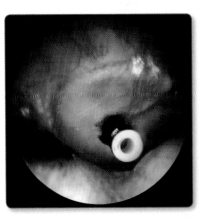

Figure 6.5 Grommet in right tympanic membrane.

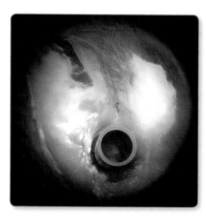

Figure 6.6 T tube in the ear (long-term grommet) with adjacent tympanosclerosis (seen as white patches).

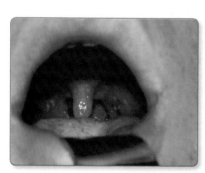

Figure 6.7 Acute tonsillitis showing classic 'white spots'.

Epidemiology

Tonsillitis is most commonly seen in children during the first 10 years of life, presumably because of a relatively immature immune system. Adenoidal hypertrophy reaches its peak between 3 and 6 years of age.

Causes

The infective causes of tonsillitis are listed in **Table 6.3**. Rarely, leukaemias and lymphomas may present with tonsillitis.

Viral causes	Bacterial causes
Adenovirus	Group A beta-haemolytic (GABH)
Epstein–Barr virus (also	*Streptococcus*
known as infectious	Non-GABH *Streptococcus*
mononucleosis, glandular	*Haemophilus influenzae*
fever)	*Staphylococcus aureus*
Parainfluenza and influenza	*Moraxella catarrhalis*

Table 6.3 Causes of tonsillitis

Pathogenesis

Most cases of tonsillitis commence with a viral infection and may progress secondarily to a bacterial infection. Although part of the immune system, the tonsils or adenoids can become the source of infection rather than a defence against it, leading to recurrent infective exacerbations and ultimately requiring removal.

Adenoids and tonsils may also become significantly hypertrophied and lead to airway compromise and obstructive sleep apnoea (OSA). OSA can have a significant impact on quality of life, with sleep disturbance leading to daytime tiredness and sleepiness affecting activities as well as causing long-term cardiovascular strain and disease.

Clinical features

The symptoms and signs of acute tonsillitis and obstructive sleep apnoea are listed in **Tables 6.4** and **6.5**, respectively.

Investigation

In most cases a diagnosis of tonsillitis can be made on clinical grounds alone.

- **Throat swabs** are not routinely required as they do not alter management, but may be considered in atypical cases or where standard therapy has failed
- **Blood tests:** in severe cases where admission to hospital is required, FBC, urea and electrolytes, and glandular fever tests are requested. With bacterial tonsillitis there is usually a

Signs	Symptoms
Enlarged erythematous tonsils with or without exudate (**Figure 6.7**)	Sore throat
Enlarged, tender cervical lymphadenopathy	Otalgia (referred pain)
Fever	Odynophagia
Trismus	Halitosis
Sometimes abdominal pain and vomiting in children	Snoring

Table 6.4 Signs and symptoms of acute tonsillitis

Signs	Symptoms
Failure to thrive/poor growth	Loud snoring (with periods of silence)
Stertor	Frequent awakening from sleep
Blocked nose	Daytime tiredness and sleepiness
Mouth breathing	Poor concentration
Enlarged tonsils	Hyperactivity in young children

Table 6.5 Signs and symptoms of obstructive sleep apnoea

raised neutrophil count, whereas with glandular fever there is usually a raised lymphocyte count. Rarely there may be a neutropenia in an immunocompromised patient or marked leucocytosis in acute leukaemia
• A **sleep study** is indicated where there is a history of sleep apnoea to ascertain the severity. In moderately severe sleep apnoea an ECG is warranted prior to adenotonsillectomy to look for signs of right heart strain.

Management

The average duration of acute tonsillitis in the community is 2–3 days; the vast majority settle with analgesia and adequate fluid intake. In those failing to resolve over 48–72 hours, or where there is clinical concern due to the severity of symptoms, antibiotics should be considered.

The Centor clinical prediction score can be used to assist the decision on whether to prescribe an antibiotic, but cannot be relied upon for a precise diagnosis.

Centor score (one point each)

- Tonsillar exudate
- Tender anterior cervical lymphadenopathy
- Fever
- Absence of cough.

A higher Centor score increases the likelihood that the patient has a group A beta-haemolytic streptococcal (GABHS) infection, and penicillin V should be prescribed (or a macrolide if there is a penicillin allergy). In acute tonsillitis, those who are unable to eat or drink, or where there is a significant systemic upset, should be admitted to hospital for observation and IV antibiotics and fluids.

If a tonsillectomy has been decided on this is usually done after an interval of 6 weeks to allow the current infective episode to resolve completely.

> **Clinical insight**
>
> Neither ampicillin nor amoxicillin should be used to treat acute tonsillitis in case the patient has glandular fever, when a generalised maculopapular rash may develop.

Indications for tonsillectomy

The commonest indication for tonsillectomy is recurrent episodes of acute tonsillitis:

- 7 or more episodes in a year
- 5 or more episodes in 2 consecutive years, or
- 3 or more episodes in 3 consecutive years.

Other indications include after an episode of quinsy, recurrent infections causing febrile convulsions, obstructive sleep apnoea and suspicion of malignancy.

> **Clinical insight**
>
> In children with a bifid uvula the soft palate should be palpated prior to adenoidectomy to rule out a submucous cleft defect. In these children the adenoid may be significantly contributing to nasopharyngeal competence, with a real chance of nasopharyngeal reflux if removed.

In the majority of children OSA is cured after adenotonsil-lectomy. Children with moderately severe OSA may require admission to ITU post-operatively and preferably should be managed in a hospital where these facilities are available. These children require overnight pulse oximetry after the operation until they are no longer desaturating at night, at which stage they can be discharged home.

Prognosis

Complications are rare with acute tonsillitis. GABHS may cause an acute exanthematous reaction with a macular rash known as scarlet fever. Tonsil infection may spread locally into the peritonsillar space, leading to peritonsillar cellulitis or abscess (less common in children). Further spread of infection can lead to a deep neck space infection. Rarely, immune-mediated disorders such as acute rheumatic fever or glomerulonephritis can result from cross-reactivity of antibodies or immune complex deposition.

Although the adenoids and tonsils are part of the immune system, there is no evidence that adenotonsillectomy is detrimental to long-term general health.

6.4 Thyroglossal cyst

Thyroglossal cysts are developmental remnants arising from incomplete obliteration of the thyroglossal duct during the migration of the thyroid gland from its origin at the tongue base (foramen caecum) to its eventual site in front of the trachea. The pyramidal lobe of the thyroid gland is in fact the caudal aspect of the duct.

Epidemiology

Thyroglossal cysts are the most common midline neck cysts. Despite being a congenital abnormality they rarely present in infants and usually present in early childhood, sometimes into adulthood. They have equal gender distribution. The vast majority occur in the midline around the hyoid bone, but they can occur within the tongue or laterally in the neck at the tip of the greater horn of the hyoid, or lower down adjacent to the thyroid gland.

Causes and pathogenesis

The aetiology is failure of obliteration of the thyroglossal duct, which transmits the thyroid diverticulum at the tuberculum impar, forming the foramen caecum at the tongue base, through the substance of the tongue and looping around the hyoid bone to its final location in the lower neck (**Figure 6.8**).

Clinical features

Most thyroglossal cysts are asymptomatic and present as a midline painless neck mass (**Figure 6.9**). Approximately 15% present as an infection (abscess) with a painful, tender, erythematous and fluctuant neck mass or a discharging sinus. Classically, they rise on protrusion of the tongue. They may

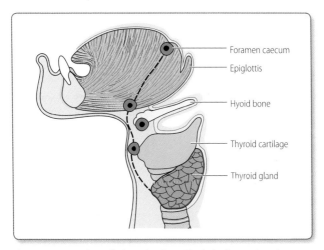

Foramen caecum

Epiglottis

Hyoid bone

Thyroid cartilage

Thyroid gland

Figure 6.8 Embryology of a thyroglossal cyst. The dashed line outlines the path of descent of the thyroid gland from the foramen caecum at the tongue base to its usual resting place in front of the trachea. The various positions for development of a thyroglossal cyst are denoted by the black dots outlined in blue.

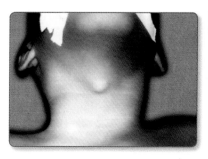

Figure 6.9 Thyroglossal cyst.

contain functioning thyroid tissue and rarely may be the only functioning thyroid tissue. Larger cysts can cause pressure symptoms such as dysphagia.

Investigation

An **ultrasound** scan of the neck is helpful to confirm the nature of the cyst as well as confirming that there is a thyroid gland in its normal location. Where there is a significant solid component to the mass an ultrasound-guided **fine-needle aspirate** is indicated. **Thyroid function tests** may be necessary when there are suggestive symptoms or unusual ultrasound findings.

Management

Asymptomatic patients may be treated with a conservative 'wait and watch' policy, depending on the age at presentation, although eventual excision is recommended. Infected cysts should not be incised and drained but rather aspiration of pus and antibiotic treatment instituted, so as to avoid fistula formation.

Surgical excision should be considered as definitive, but recurrence rates vary widely depending on the extent of surgery. It is now accepted that a wide excision of the cyst, the tract, the mid-third of the hyoid and a wedge of tongue (modified Sistrunk's procedure) be performed. This helps reduce recurrence rates considerably. Complications of the surgery include keloid scarring in susceptible individuals, recurrence, sinus/fistula formation, damage to the hypoglossal nerve, infection and bleeding from the tongue base. A drain is therefore placed to reduce collection of blood postoperatively. The specimen should be sent for histological analysis.

Prognosis

Recurrence of thyroglossal cysts varies widely (20–30%) depending on the extent of surgery, and also whether the operation was a revision case. A modified Sistrunk's procedure, however, has an excellent prognosis. Finally, it is a very rare possibility that a finding of carcinoma be made. In this case, the patient is referred to a thyroid oncologist for further management.

6.5 Paediatric hearing loss

Hearing is essential for normal speech development, and if left untreated can have a devastating effect on child's social interactions and school performance. Therefore, a prompt diagnosis and timely management of the hearing loss and any possible associated disabilities is crucial.

Epidemiology

Severe to profound congenital sensorineural hearing loss (SNHL) occurs in 1 in every 1000 live births in the UK. By school entry age the incidence has almost doubled.

Causes

Hearing loss can be sensorineural, conductive or mixed. Its aetiology can be classified as hereditary or acquired and also categorised by the time of onset into prenatal, perinatal and postnatal, as shown in **Table 6.6**.

Stage	Causes
Prenatal	• Syndromic, e.g. Usher's, Waardenburg's • Non-syndromic, e.g. Connexin 26 • Intrauterine infections, e.g. TORCH (*Toxoplasma gondii*, other viruses*, rubella, cytomegalovirus, herpes simplex) • Ototoxic agents *Hepatitis B, coxsackievirus, syphilis, varicella zoster, HIV, parvovirus B19
Perinatal	• Prematurity • Birth weight <1.5 kg • Hypoxia • Hyperbilirubinaemia • Apgar score <4 at 1 minute
Postnatal	• Meningitis • Otitis media (acute and chronic) • Otitis media with effusion

Table 6.6 Causes of paediatric hearing loss

Investigation
Identification of hearing loss
Paediatric hearing loss can be identified through targeted, universal, opportunistic or preschool screening.

- **Targeted screening** aims at neonates with three major risk factors, including a positive family history of SNHL, craniofacial abnormalities and admission to a neonatal intensive care. Targeted screening can identify up to 70% of cases
- **Universal screening** was introduced in the UK in 2005 to raise the detection rate. It is routine practice to perform transient otoacoustic emission (TOAE) testing in neonates in most hospitals
- **Opportunistic hearing screening** takes place when a child is being presented to the otolaryngologist for other reasons
- **Pre-school screening** aims to detect hearing loss missed by other screening methods, as well as in those who develop hearing impairment later in childhood.

Audiological tests

Audiological tests can be classified based on different age groups, which usually correspond to developmental status. Tests may be modified for children with developmental delay. Age-appropriate hearing tests are listed in **Table 6.7**.

Transient otoacoustic emission (TOAE)   The TOAE test is a pass or fail inner ear test that assesses the presence of a cochlear outer hair cell (OHC) response, and can be used in all age groups. The sensitivity of the test is high, therefore it is used in universal neonatal hearing screening. It has a relatively low specificity as the response may be absent in conditions such as otitis media with effusion.

Auditory brainstem response (ABR) This test assesses the auditory pathway from cochlea to cortex and can predict the hearing threshold between 2 and 4 kHz. Typically, ABR shows five waveforms, each corresponding to an anatomical location (and giving the acronym *E COLI*):
- **E**ighth nerve action potential
- **C**ochlear nuclei
- **O**livary (superior) complex
- **L**ateral lemniscus
- **I**nferior colliculus.

Age group	Appropriate hearing tests
Birth – 6 months	• Transient otoacoustic emissions (TOAE) • Auditory brainstem response (ABR) • Tympanometry
6 – 24 months	• Distraction testing (DT) • Visual reinforcement audiometry (VRA)
24 months – 4 years	• Play audiometry • Speech audiometry
>4 years	• Pure tone audiogram (PTA)

Table 6.7 Age-appropriate hearing tests

Maturation and the presence of all five waveforms occur by 4 weeks of age. In the universal screening, neonates who fail TOAE will require an ABR test.

Tympanometry Tympanometry is a quick and objective test that indirectly assesses middle ear function. It is not a hearing test but rather a measure of impedance at the tympanic membrane (see p. 63).

Visual reinforcement audiometry (VRA) This takes place in a 'soundproof' environment:
- The child sits on the parent's lap, facing a tester, who will attract the child's attention
- A second tester behind a one-way mirror is in charge of presenting sound stimuli via speakers or headphones
- A positive response with a correct head-turn towards the noise is rewarded by a light flashing or a toy moving.

Distraction test Used by health visitors in children between 6–9 months of age, the distraction test involves the baby turning its head to an ear-level sound (commonly a high-frequency rattle) presented outside the visual field from behind.

Play audiometry Play audiometry is a performance test where the child is conditioned to perform certain tasks in response to a pure tone. Therefore, it is essential that child is able to follow simple commands.

Speech audiometry An example of speech audiometry is the McCormick toy test, which demands an appropriate level

---

Clinical insight

Significant coexisting disability is present in about 30% of children with significant sensorineural hearing loss. For example:
- **Alport's** and **branchio-oto-renal syndromes** - renal impairment
- **Stickler and Usher syndromes** - visual impairment
- **Pendred syndrome** - thyroid dysfunction
- **Jervell–Lange–Neilson syndrome** - prolonged Q-T intervals on ECG.

It is essential to identify, evaluate and manage these disabilities. Based on the history and examination, further tests may be required as well as referral to the appropriate specialist.

of language development. This test consists of seven pairs of toys matched to contain the same sound, such as key/tree and cup/duck. In a 'soundproof' environment the child is asked to point to a toy.

Pure tone audiogram Pure tone audiography can be performed on a child from 4 to 5 years of age (p. 62).

Management
When planning management it is important to recognise the impact that prolonged hearing loss can have on a child's development and social interactions. Remediable causes should be treated early and where necessary rehabilitation and hearing aids should be offered.

6.6 Congenital ear deformities
Congenital defects of the pinna and external ear canal can be classified into genetic, environmental or multifactorial aetiologies. A detailed knowledge of the embryological development of the ear is beyond the scope of this book, but is useful in understanding these conditions.

This chapter limits discussion to the more commonly encountered congenital external ear defects:
- Prominent ears (**Figure 6.10**)
- Preauricular abnormalities, e.g. abscess (**Figure 6.11**)
- Microtia (**Figure 6.12**).

Epidemiology
- Prominent ears are relatively common, with a prevalence of 5%, and they tend to be bilateral
- Preauricular sinuses or tags occur in 0.5% of the general population, and again are commonly bilateral
- Microtia occurs in 1 in 6000 births, is three times more common in males and is bilateral in 10%.

Causes and pathogenesis
In most cases the cause is unknown.

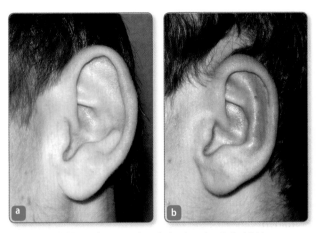

Figure 6.10 (a) Protruding ear with underdeveloped antihelical fold. (b) Antihelical fold restored after pinnaplasty surgery.

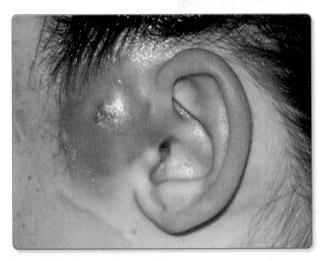

Figure 6.11 Left preauricular sinus and abscess.

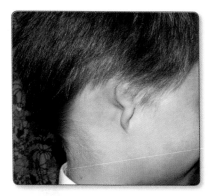

Figure 6.12 Right microtia

Prominent ears Protruding ears tend to run in families, implying a strong genetic component, although birth trauma has also been implicated.

Preauricular sinuses or tags Preauricular sinuses are thought to be the result of incomplete fusion of the hillocks of His of the first and second branchial arches during embryogenesis. They are inherited in a variable and reduced-penetrant autosomal dominant pattern.

Microtia Certain teratogenic compounds, such as isotretinoin and thalidomide, cause hypoplasia of the ear.

Syndromes As the ear (external and middle) is derived from the first two branchial arches and their associated grooves and pouches, a malformed pinna and/or external ear canal often acts as a marker for underlying middle ear defects. There may also be features of syndromes intimately related to developmental failure of these arches, e.g. Goldenhar's, branchio-oto-renal and Treacher–Collins syndromes. All children presenting with defects in the development of the external ear should therefore undergo a thorough audiological assessment, careful examination of both sides of the head and neck, and a systemic examination.

Clinical features

The clinical features of the more common congenital defects are described in **Table 6.8**.

Clinical insight

Beware of a pit/cyst in the preauricular region presenting below the level of the tragus, nearer the jaw line, which implies a first branchial cleft anomaly, as does a fistula into the external auditory canal. If suspected, an MRI scan may be helpful to delineate the extent of the lesion and its intimate relationship to the facial nerve.

Investigation

The investigations of the more common congenital defects are described in **Table 6.9**.

Management

Prominent ears If protruding ears are noticed soon after birth, growth of the pinna may be redirected by splinting the ears back for 6 months, although this has variable success.

Surgery remains the definitive option (see **Figure 6.10b**) and is ideally performed just before school age, to obviate teasing and to ensure compliance with postoperative care. Pinnaplasty

Condition	Clinical features
Preauricular sinus	• A 'pit' in the skin anterior to the root of the helix, above the level of the tragus • Can initially present as tender fluctuant abscess in the preauricular region (**Figure 6.11**)
Protruding ear	• Prominence is usually caused by an absent antihelical fold. • May be associated deep conchal bowl ('unfolded' appearance)
Microtia	• Extent of the abnormality varies from a mild deformity with an anatomically intact but slightly smaller ear, to cases with significant morphological abnormalities (**Figure 6.12**) • With classic 'peanut' ear only an anteriorly placed lobule remnant remains • The EAC may be narrow or even absent

Table 6.8 Clinical features of common congenital ear defects

Condition	Investigations
Preauricular sinus	Clinical diagnosis; however, a preauricular abscess should have pus sent for microbiological analysis
Protruding ear	Standardised photography essential for preoperative counselling and evaluation of surgery (**Figure 6.10**)
Microtia	Full paediatric audiological assessment as often a conductive hearing loss on the affected side High-resolution CT scan of the temporal bones when considering surgery for concurrent EAC/middle ear defects

Table 6.9 Investigations for common congenital ear defects

surgery will be tailored to the ear, but usually comprises excision of an ellipse of postauricular skin, cartilage scoring, and carefully tensioned sutures to maintain the new position of the pinna. A headband is worn for a week afterwards and then at night for a month or so.

Preauricular sinuses or tags
Preauricular sinuses may be left alone if asymptomatic. An acute abscess (**Figure 6.11**) should be aspirated with a needle and the patient given a course of broad-spectrum antibiotic (e.g. co-amoxiclav).

> **Clinical insight**
>
> After pinnaplasty for protruding ears, increasing pain should alert you to the possibility of haematoma or abscess formation. The head bandage should be removed and the wound inspected.

Once the infection/inflammation has settled, a wider, more complete surgical excision will minimise scar formation and recurrence. It is important to differentiate a complicated pre-auricular sinus from a first branchial cleft anomaly (see above). In the latter, the surgical management is significantly more difficult as the facial nerve is intimately involved.

Microtia Surgical reconstruction of the severely microtic, de-formed pinna is technically difficult and should be performed in a specialist centre. It comprises a multistage procedure us-ing the child's rib cartilage, which is shaped into a neo pinna.

Clinical insight

There is a significant risk to the facial nerve from reconstructive surgery for congenital atresia of the external acoustic meatus. There has been a move away from this surgery to good auditory rehabilitation using bone-anchored hearing aids.

The alternative is to create a prosthetic pinna based on the good ear, which may be clipped on to the head via a surgically integrated (into the bony skull) titanium abutment. This may be a more cosmetically acceptable solution for some families.

A bone-conducting or bone-anchored hearing aid is often the more satisfactory option to address the accompanying conductive hearing loss.

Careful **counselling** and long-term follow-up are very important in the management of microtia.

Prognosis

Once a confident diagnosis has been made, symptomatic preauricular sinuses are successfully treated by wide local excision.

Conservative management of protruding ears is often unsuccessful and the mainstay of management is necessarily surgical. The cosmetic success will vary depending on the anatomy of the individual pinna and the technical expertise of the surgeon. The latter is crucial in microtia surgery, where there have been significant recent surgical advances in pinna reconstruction. Nevertheless, in severe cases it may be impossible to match the patient's expectations.

6.7 The catarrhal child

Description

Catarrh is defined as fluid flowing from a mucous membrane. The 'catarrhal child' shows an excessive response from the nasal mucous membranes to various factors in what is essentially paediatric rhinosinusitis. These children present with persistent rhinorrhoea or nasal discharge.

Epidemiology

More than 50% of children seen in primary care present with upper respiratory symptoms, commonly those between 3 and

8 years of age. It is often worse in the winter, when such infections are more common.

Causes

The main causal factors are:
- frequent URTIs
- the child's relatively immature immune system
- the prevalence of allergic rhinitis and adenoidal hypertrophy.

It is interesting to note that children between the ages of 2 and 5 have on average eight episodes of URTI per year. These are caused by viruses, leading to a serous nasal discharge, which then becomes mucopurulent and resolves generally over 10 days. However, mucociliary clearance is affected for 4–6 weeks after a viral URTI, and can be further hampered by another URTI.

Allergic rhinitis (see p. 124) affects one in four children and can lead to persistent rhinorrhoea. Adenoidal hypertrophy is common in young children up to the age of 8 and can cause obstruction of the postnasal space, leading to nasal blockage and discharge.

Other factors that may play a role are:
- anatomical abnormalities (e.g. septal deviation, choanal stenosis and atresia)
- mucosal abnormalities (Young's syndrome, Kartagener's syndrome, cystic fibrosis)
- immunological deficiencies (e.g. IgG subclass deficiency).

Pathogenesis

Increased nasal activity with excessive mucus production is essentially hypersecretion of the mucus-secreting glands. Mucus glycoproteins are secreted by goblet cells and by serous and mucous glandular cells in the submucosal glands. The secretory component is made by the serous cells in the seromucous glands.

Clinical features

In a baby symptoms include:
- snuffles
- snoring

- mouth breathing
- feeding difficulties
- cough
- sleep disturbance.

In an older child:

- rhinorrhoea
- nasal discharge
- nasal obstruction
- sneezing
- bad breath
- hyposmia.

Examination may reveal a runny nose and breathing through an open mouth. Nasal airflow and patency can be simply demonstrated by holding a metal tongue depressor under the nose and observing the misting pattern. The colour of any secretions should be noted, as clear discharge may suggest the early stages of a viral infection or allergic rhinitis, whereas a greenish-yellow purulent discharge may suggest a bacterial infection. The inferior nasal turbinates may be oedematous and pale (allergic rhinitis) or congested and erythematous (acute infection). Nasal polyps are rarely seen in children and should alert one to the possibility of cystic fibrosis.

Nasal endoscopy is not routinely used in children and is generally difficult in children under 6 years of age.

Investigation

In the vast majority of cases investigations are not necessary. Those to consider are listed in **Table 6.10**.

Clinical insight

Children with allergic rhinitis have an increased chance of having asthma, and vice versa, which should prompt a search for both conditions.

Management

There is usually considerable parental anxiety and it is important to reassure parents that in the vast majority the child's symptoms will abate with age. Management principles include:

- Empirical treatment includes encouraging nose-blowing to clear secretions and the use of saline sprays or douches,

Investigation	Description
Allergy test	> 5 years of age: skin prick test < 5 years: IgE blood test for common inhalant allergens
Blood tests	Full blood count Total immunoglobins Immunoglobulin subclasses
Plain radiography	Plain sinus radiographs show changes in 30–50% of asymptomatic children May be indicated in the presence of an opaque foreign body or acute sinusitis where drainage is being considered Postnasal space radiographs may help demonstrate adenoidal hypertrophy
CT scan of sinuses	Not routine: radiation exposure, high incidence of 'normal' mucosal changes and need for sedation Can help tumour diagnosis or pre-op assessment
MRI scan of sinuses	May require sedation and prevalence of incidental changes is high, so should be restricted for investigation of nasal masses

Table 6.10 Investigations to consider with persistent nasal discharge in a child

as well as a short course of a nasal decongestant and topical steroid
- With allergic rhinitis, an oral or topical antihistamine and topical steroid nasal spray with specific allergen avoidance is beneficial
- Antibiotics have shown to be effective in the short to medium term, although symptoms tend to recur in the longer term. A long-term (6–12 weeks) once-daily low-dose macrolide (e.g. clarithromycin) may be useful
- Surgery is rarely indicated and may involve adenoidectomy and submucous diathermy to the inferior turbinates.

Clinical insight

Failure to demonstrate nasal patency, e.g. by absent misting on a cold metal tongue depressor, should alert one to the possibility of choanal atresia. Although bilateral cases present at birth as an airway emergency, unilateral cases can go unrecognised for several years and usually present with nasal discharge.

Prognosis

Studies of the natural history of persistent rhinorrhoea in children unresponsive to medical treatment show that 95% resolve spontaneously by the age of 7.

6.8 Foreign bodies in the ear, nose and throat

Description

Children often present with foreign bodies in the ear and nose, but also more rarely and dangerously in the throat. Most foreign bodies in the ear and nose include inorganic material such as plastic toys and beads, stones, and organic substances such as food, cotton bud tips, paper, sponge, wood, feathers etc. Occasionally watch batteries are inserted which leak caustic substances, causing rapid and irreversible erosion of the surrounding tissue.

Epidemiology

Foreign bodies in the ear, nose and throat present at different ages depending on the site, but can be seen and should be suspected in any age group. If missed in childhood or in patients with psychiatric illness they may not present until adulthood (e.g. rhinoliths). The majority of ear foreign bodies present in children aged 7 or under. Nasal foreign bodies are commonest between 2 and 5 years of age.

Causes and pathogenesis

In the vast majority of children the cause is fairly obvious, although child neglect/abuse should be considered if the type of foreign body is uncharacteristic for the age group, or if clinical examination raises other suspicions.

Clinical features

In children foreign bodies are classified by whether they are organic or inorganic and whether they are in the ear, nose or upper aerodigestive tract:

- Ear: foreign bodies in the ear are often asymptomatic, although they can present with pain, bleeding, discharge and hearing loss
- Nose: those in the nose often present with unilateral foul-smelling discharge, epistaxis and rhinorrhoea. Occasionally they can be aspirated
- Throat: foreign bodies in the larynx and trachea can be asymptomatic, but more often present with stridor, cough, wheeze and respiratory difficulty. Rarely, there is sudden loss of the airway and respiratory arrest. Fish bones tend to lodge in the tonsil, tongue base or valecculla.

Investigation

Anteroposterior and lateral neck and chest **radiographs** are essential in distinguishing the location of the foreign body in the pharynx/upper oesophagus and larynx. Occasionally a lateral skull radiograph can help distinguish a radio-opaque foreign body such as a watch battery in the nose/postnasal space.

Management

Most foreign bodies in the ear, nose and throat are easily removed with no long-term sequelae. Potential exceptions include a corroding watch battery, as it has the potential to cause nasal septal perforation and collapse, external acoustic meatal stenosis and tympanic membrane perforation or pharyngeal/oesophageal stricture.

> ### Clinical insight
>
> - The use of irrigation (ear syringing) to remove an aural foreign body is contraindicated for hydrophilic items such as peas, beans and other vegetable matter, which may expand further in the presence of liquid
> - Spherical objects are best removed with the aid of a Jobson Horne probe with the end gently bent at about 5 mm from the tip. The probe is passed above and behind the foreign body and raked forwards.

The most important adage for foreign body removal from the ear or nose in children is that 'the first attempt is the best attempt'. Repeated attempts at removal cause trauma, fear and loss of confidence from the child and parents. Children should be securely restrained by their parents/guardians in a child-friendly environment with good access to illumination and suction. After a failed attempt to remove a foreign body from the ear or nose in a young child, a general anaesthetic is usually required to prevent further distress.

Foreign bodies in the ear or nose Most inorganic foreign bodies in the ear (e.g. beads) cause little harm and can be removed easily in the outpatient setting or at the next available theatre list. Organic material can decompose and cause otitis externa, bleeding and deafness (conductive loss); insects should be drowned with olive oil. Nasal foreign bodies are usually removed earlier because of the potential risk of aspiration, and batteries should be removed with particular urgency.

Foreign bodies in the throat These invariably involve a multidisciplinary approach with a trained paediatric anaesthetist familiar with ventilating bronchoscopy. Foreign bodies at the level of the cricopharyngeus should be removed early under general anaesthesia (**Figure 6.13**). Similarly, sharp bones represent an urgent presentation as there is a risk of perforation and infection. Other smooth objects such as coins that have migrated beyond the pharynx into the oesophagus usually pass spontaneously, and can therefore be treated conservatively.

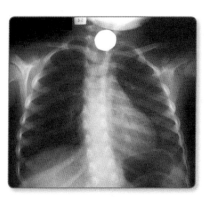

Figure 6.13 Chest radiograph showing a coin at the level of the upper oesophagus.

Prognosis

In the vast majority of cases, once the foreign body has been removed the child makes a full recovery. Long-term sequelae can result from excessive tissue damage and scarring from alkaline battery leakage. Rarely an emergency cricothyroidotomy may be required when the larynx has been obstructed. This involves making an incision through the cricothyroid membrane and inserting a suitable airway.

6.9 Paediatric upper airway disorders

Description

Upper airway compromise gives rise to turbulent airflow and noisy breathing, with stertor or stridor:

- **Stertor** is noisy breathing caused by partial obstruction of the airway above the level of the larynx. It resembles a 'snoring' sound, lower in pitch than stridor, which is a harsher sound
- **Stridor** is noisy breathing caused by partial obstruction of the airway at the level of the larynx or trachea and may occur on inspiration, expiration or both.

Epidemiology

The commonest cause of paediatric stridor is croup (acute laryngotracheobronchitis), which accounts for 90% of cases. Laryngomalacia is the commonest neonatal cause.

Causes and pathogenesis

Causes of upper airway disorders can be congenital or acquired, and according to the site of obstruction (oral, nasal, pharyngeal, laryngeal and tracheal). For the purposes of this book the more common causes are listed in **Table 6.11**.

Clinical features

History It is important to establish the onset of the noisy breathing:

- rapid onset (this may signify an inhaled foreign body or an allergic reaction)

Cause	Description
Choanal atresia	Persistence of bony/ membranous plate blocking the posterior nares. Bilateral presents at birth with upper airway obstruction as neonates are obligate nose breathers
Adenotonsillar hypertrophy	Adenotonsillar enlargement can lead to obstruction, stertor and obstructive sleep apnoea
Micrognathia or macroglossia	A small jaw (e.g. Pierre Robin sequence) or enlarged tongue can give rise to stertor
Retropharyngeal abscess	Suppuration of retropharyngeal lymph nodes from infected tonsils, teeth, pharynx, sinuses or foreign body Can expand rapidly
Foreign bodies	Most common in children under 3 years Present with noisy breathing and (if at laryngeal level) cough/choking
Lymphovascular malformations	Anomaly of angiovascular or lymphovascular structures which can grow to considerable size and compromise the upper airway
Croup	Laryngotracheobronchitis, usually triggered by an acute viral infection Inspiratory stridor is accompanied by a harsh cough
Laryngomalacia	A 'floppy larynx' due to laryngeal immaturity. Stridor is caused by an excessive indrawing of the epiglottis upon inspiration. Usually self-limiting
Epiglottitis	Acute infection of the supraglottic larynx usually caused by *Haemophilus influenzae B*
Vocal fold palsy	In congenital palsy 50% are unilateral and 50% recover spontaneously. Bilateral palsy presents with stridor
Respiratory papillomatosis	Multiple papillomas (viral warts) in the upper airway caused by the human papillomavirus (type 6 and 11) **(Figure 6.14)**
Subglottic stenosis	Narrowing of the subglottis can be congenital or acquired (the majority are caused by endotracheal intubation)
Subglottic haemangioma	The most common neoplasm of the infant airway; 50% also have an associated cutaneous haemangioma

Contd...

Contd...

Cause	Description
Vascular ring	Abnormal development of the great vessels in the chest surrounding and compressing the trachea and oesophagus, producing biphasic stridor and feeding difficulties
Tracheomalacia	Softening of the tracheal rings, which may be intrinsically weak or acquired (usually due to external compression by an abnormal great vessel)

Table 6.11 Causes of paediatric upper airway compromise

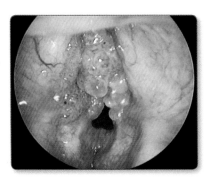

Figure 6.14 An endoscopic view of the larynx showing respiratory papillomatosis.

- onset from birth (a congenital cause)
- onset after the first week of life (laryngomalacia or subglottic haemangioma)
- onset after a febrile illness (infection).

The noisy breathing may be exacerbated by feeding and crying or lying supine (laryngomalacia). There may be an associated abnormal cry indicative of a congenital laryngeal web or recurrent laryngeal nerve palsy, or dysphonia in an older child with laryngeal papillomatosis. Worsening stridor after feeding could indicate aspiration or a fistula. The latter may give rise to post-feeding cyanotic episodes. Recurrent cyanotic attacks may indicate tracheomalacia.

The neonatal history is particularly important:

- Neonatal intubation is the commonest cause of acquired subglottic cysts and stenosis
- Cardiac surgery (e.g. patent ductus arteriosus ligation) commonly causes (temporary) left recurrent laryngeal nerve palsy
- Traumatic birth may also result in laryngeal nerve damage.

Examination   Examine for signs of respiratory distress. Look for:

- stertor
- stridor
- cough and dysphonia
- drooling
- pallor
- cyanosis
- tachypnoea
- nasal flaring
- tracheal tug
- intercostal recession.

A 'toxic' appearance with an altered mental state indicates impending respiratory failure. Chronic obstruction may lead to permanent chest deformities, such as pectus carinatum or Harrison's sulci. Oral examination and invasive manoeuvres such as intravenous cannulation should not be performed until the child is in an environment with personnel and facilities to instigate swift airway intervention. Look also for cutaneous haemangioma and craniofacial anomalies, which may give further clues to the aetiology.

> **Clinical insight**
>
> A child's weight is a sensitive marker for chronic airway compromise owing to the extra calories used for laboured breathing. Poor progress on growth charts and failure to thrive may indicate the need for active intervention (e.g. surgical release of the epiglottis (aryepiglottoplasty) for laryngomalacia).

Investigation

Oxygen saturation should be continuously monitored. However, it should be remembered that considerable airway obstruction can occur without desaturation as the child works hard to overcome the obstruction.

Plain chest and lateral soft tissue neck radiographs may be useful, but should be deferred until an imminently compromised airway has been secured.

Laryngotracheobronchoscopy under general anaesthesia may be required for a definitive diagnosis and for management. High-resolution imaging modalities (CT/MRI) may also be required, but again these should be performed only once the airway has been secured.

Management

General principles for managing any upper airway emergency include:

- Sit the child upright and commence high-flow humidified oxygen via a facemask
- Administer an adrenaline nebuliser (1 mL 1:1000 adrenaline in 4 mL normal saline)
- Commence systemic steroids (0.1–0.2 mg/kg dexamethasone orally, or intravenously if access has already been obtained).

These manoeuvres will buy time until the airway is definitely secured. Mobilise senior colleagues in anaesthetics, ENT and paediatrics. Recognise impending airway failure and transfer the child to a safe environment, ideally into a theatre, where nursing staff are able to swiftly locate and mobilise specialist equipment. The child may need a nasopharyngeal airway and manual ventilation with a bag and mask prior to attempted endotracheal intubation. If the latter is deemed a possibility, then a senior ENT surgeon should be scrubbed and ready with open rigid bronchoscopy and tracheostomy sets.

Definitive investigations and management can be commenced after the airway is secured.

Prognosis

Owing to advances in anaesthesia and paediatric endoscopy, intubation is rarely unsuccessful in a way that would necessitate emergency tracheostomy.

Appendix

NICE guidelines on surgical management of paediatric otitis media with effusion

An algorithm summarising the NICE 2008 guidelines for the surgical management of paediatric otitis media with effusion is shown on the following two pages. The full guideline, developed by the UK's National Collaborating Centre for Women's and Children's Health, is available at http://guidance.nice.org.uk/CG60.

NICE 2008 guideline on the surgical management of paediatric otitis media with effusion. With permission from NICE clinical guideline 60. Surgical management of otitis media with effusion in children. Quick reference guide. London: NICE, 2008.

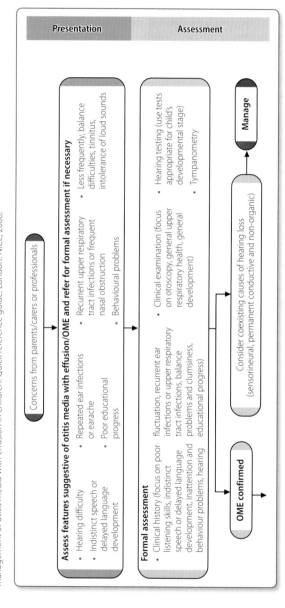

Presentation

Assessment

Concerns from parents/carers or professionals

Assess features suggestive of otitis media with effusion/OME and refer for formal assessment if necessary

- Hearing difficulty
- Indistinct speech or delayed language development
- Repeated ear infections or earache
- Poor educational progress
- Recurrent upper respiratory tract infections or frequent nasal obstruction
- Behavioural problems
- Less frequently, balance difficulties, tinnitus, intolerance of loud sounds

Formal assessment

- Clinical history (focus on poor listening skills, indistinct speech or delayed language development, inattention and behaviour problems, hearing fluctuation, recurrent ear infections or upper respiratory tract infections, balance problems and clumsiness, educational progress)
- Clinical examination (focus on otoscopy, general upper respiratory health, general development)
- Hearing testing (use tests appropriate for child's developmental stage)
- Tympanometry

Consider coexisting causes of hearing loss (sensorineural, permanent conductive and non-organic)

OME confirmed

Manage

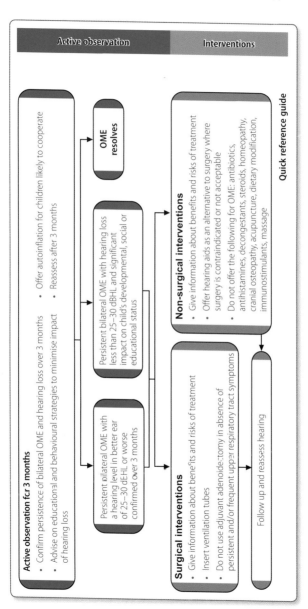

Active observation | **Interventions**

Active observation for 3 months
- Confirm persistence of bilateral OME and hearing loss over 3 months
- Advise on educational and behavioural strategies to minimise impact of hearing loss
- Offer autoinflation for children likely to cooperate
- Reassess after 3 months

OME resolves

Persistent bilateral OME with a hearing level in better ear of 25–30 dEHL or worse confirmed over 3 months

Persistent bilateral OME with hearing loss less than 25–30 dBHL and significant impact on child's developmental, social or educational status

Surgical interventions
- Give information about benefits and risks of treatment
- Insert ventilation tubes
- Do not use adjuvant adenoidectomy in absence of persistent and/or frequent upper respiratory tract symptoms

Non-surgical interventions
- Give information about benefits and risks of treatment
- Offer hearing aids as an alternative to surgery where surgery is contraindicated or not acceptable
- Do not offer the following for OME: antibiotics, antihistamines, decongestants, steroids, homeopathy, cranial osteopathy, acupuncture, dietary modification, immunostimulants, massage

Follow up and reassess hearing

Quick reference guide

Index

Note: Page numbers in **bold** or *italic* refer to tables or figures respectively.